# POCKET GUIDE TO
# Body CT Differential Diagnosis

## With contributions from

### Dennis M. Balfe, M.D.
Professor and Chief of Gastrointestinal Radiology
Mallinckrodt Institute of Radiology
Washington University School of Medicine, St. Louis, Missouri

### Matthew J. Fleishman, M.D.
Radiology Imaging Associates
Englewood, Colorado

### David S. Gierada, M.D.
Assistant Professor of Radiology, Chest Section
Mallinckrodt Institute of Radiology
Washington University School of Medicine, St. Louis, Missouri

### Louis A. Gilula, M.D.
Professor and Chief of Musculoskeletal Radiology
Mallinckrodt Institute of Radiology
Washington University School of Medicine, St. Louis, Missouri

### Christopher J. Gordon, M.D.
Clinical Instructor of Radiology, Chest Section
Mallinckrodt Institute of Radiology
Washington University School of Medicine, St. Louis, Missouri

### Fernando R. Gutierrez, M.D.
Associate Professor and Director of Cardiac Radiology
Mallinckrodt Institute of Radiology
Washington University School of Medicine, St. Louis, Missouri

### Cary L. Siegel, M.D.
Assistant Professor and Chief of Genitourinary Radiology
Mallinckrodt Institute of Radiology
Washington University School of Medicine, St. Louis, Missouri

### Franz J. Wippold II, M.D.
Associate Professor of Radiology, Neuroradiology Section
Mallinckrodt Institute of Radiology
Washington University School of Medicine, St. Louis, Missouri
and
Clinical Associate Professor of Radiology and Nuclear Medicine
Uniformed Services University of the Health Sciences, Bethesda, Maryland

# POCKET GUIDE TO
# Body CT Differential Diagnosis

**Richard M. Slone, M.D.**
Assistant Professor of Radiology
Thoracic Imaging and Body CT
Mallinckrodt Institute of Radiology
Washington University School of Medicine
St. Louis, Missouri

**Andrew J. Fisher, M.D.**
Assistant Professor of Radiology
Director of Emergency and Trauma Radiology
Division of Musculoskeletal Radiology
Mallinckrodt Institute of Radiology
Washington University School of Medicine
St. Louis, Missouri

# McGraw-Hill
HEALTH PROFESSIONS DIVISION

*New York   St. Louis   San Francisco   Auckland   Bogotá
Caracas   Lisbon   London   Madrid   Mexico City   Milan   Montreal
New Delhi   San Juan   Singapore   Sydney   Tokyo   Toronto*

# *McGraw-Hill*

*A Division of The **McGraw·Hill** Companies*

**Pocket Guide to Body CT
Differential Diagnosis**

Copyright © 1999 by *The **McGraw-Hill** Companies,* Inc. All rights reserved. Printed in the United States of America. Except as permitted under the United States Copyright Act of 1976, no part of this publication may be reproduced or distributed in any form or by any means, or stored in a data base or retrieval system, without the prior permission of the publisher.

1234567890   DOCDOC   998

ISBN   0-07-134435-7

This book was set in Times Roman by Bi-Comp, Inc.
The editors were James Morgan III and Muza Navrozov.
The production supervisor was Catherine H. Saggese.
The cover was designed by Li Chen Chang/Pinpoint Design.
The index was prepared by Jerry Ralya.
R. R. Donnelley & Sons Company was printer and binder.

This book is printed on acid-free paper.

**Library of Congress Cataloging-in-Publication Data**

Slone, Richard M.
Pocket guide to body CT differential diagnosis/Richard M. Slone & Andrew J. Fisher.
   p.   cm.
   Includes bibliographical references.
   ISBN 0-07-134435-7
   1. Tomography—Handbooks, manuals, etc.   2. Diagnosis,
Differential—Handbooks, manuals, etc.   I. Fisher, Andrew J.
II. Title.
   [DNLM:   1. Tomography, X-Ray Computed handbooks.   2. Diagnosis,
Differential handbooks.   WN 39S634b   1999]
RC78.7.T6S58   1999
616.07'57—dc21
DNLM/DLC
for Library of Congress

To Logan Alexander Slone
RMS

To Tanya—Without you, this never would have happened
AJF

## NOTICE

Medicine is an ever-changing science. As new research and clinical experience broaden our knowledge, changes in treatment and drug therapy are required. The editors and the publisher of this work have checked with sources believed to be reliable in their efforts to provide information that is complete and generally in accord with the standards accepted at the time of publication. However, in view of the possibility of human error or changes in medical sciences, neither the editors nor the publisher nor any other party who has been involved in the preparation or publication of this work warrants that the information contained herein is in every respect accurate or complete, and they are not responsible for any errors or omissions or for the results obtained from use of such information. Readers are encouraged to confirm the information contained herein with other sources. For example and in particular, readers are advised to check the product information sheet included in the package of each drug they plan to administer to be certain that the information contained in this book is accurate and that changes have not been made in the recommended dose or in the contraindications for administration. This recommendation is of particular importance in connection with new or infrequently used drugs.

# CONTENTS

*Preface* xiii
*Acronyms* xv

**Fleishman's 10 Rules of Boardmanship** 1

**ADENOPATHY** 3
Normal lymph node sizes 4
Calcified lymph nodes 5
Low-attenuation adenopathy 7
Hypervascular lymph nodes 9

**LOWER NECK AND TRACHEA** 11
Neck mass 12
Cystic neck mass 15
Thoracic inlet or superior mediastinal mass 17
Thyroid lesion 18
Enlarged parotid gland 20
Narrowed larynx 22
Tracheal narrowing 23
Tracheal enlargement 26
Tracheal or endobronchial mass 27

**LUNG** 29
**Global Pulmonary Patterns** 30
Diffuse lung disease 30
Diffuse interstitial lung disease with normal or increased
   lung volumes 38
Peripheral lung disease 39
Perihilar lung disease 41

## CONTENTS

Upper lung disease — 43
Lower lung disease — 45
Hyperlucent lung — 48
Asymmetric lung size — 50
Atelectasis and pulmonary collapse — 51
Bronchiectasis — 52

**Pulmonary Cysts and Nodules** — 54
Solitary pulmonary nodule — 54
Solitary pulmonary mass — 59
Peripheral pulmonary mass — 63
Cavitary lung lesion — 65
Multiple lucent lesions or cysts — 69
Multiple well-defined pulmonary nodules — 72
Multiple ill-defined pulmonary nodules — 76
Multiple cavitary nodules — 79
Tiny nodules — 82
Pulmonary nodules with adenopathy — 85
Calcified pulmonary nodules — 86

**Interstitial Lung Disease** — 88
Diffuse interstitial lung disease — 88
Nodular interstitial disease — 91
Diffuse interstitial disease with pleural effusion — 95
Diffuse interstitial disease with adenopathy — 96

**Airspace Disease** — 98
Focal or multifocal consolidation — 98
Nodular airspace disease — 102
Chronic consolidation — 104
Diffuse pulmonary consolidation — 107
Pulmonary hemorrhage — 110

**HRCT Patterns** — 112
ground-glass opacities — 112
Septal thickening — 115
Peribronchovascular interstitial thickening — 117
Small nodular opacities — 119
Small nodule distribution on HRCT — 123

**PLEURA** — 127
Pneumothorax — 128
Types of pleural fluid — 131
Unilateral pleural effusion — 135
Bilateral pleural effusions — 138

CONTENTS ix

Pleural effusion with cardiomegaly ... 140
Pleural thickening ... 142
Pleural calcifications ... 143
Pleural mass ... 144
Multiple pleural masses ... 146
Extrapleural lesion ... 148

## MEDIASTINUM AND HILA ... 149
Pneumomediastinum ... 150
Unilateral hilar enlargement ... 151
Bilateral hilar enlargement ... 153
Cardiophrenic angle mass ... 155
Anterior mediastinal mass ... 157
Middle mediastinal mass ... 160
Posterior mediastinal mass ... 165
Low-attenuation mediastinal mass ... 168

## CARDIAC AND VASCULAR ... 171
Cardiomegaly ... 172
Cardiac mass ... 175
Pericardial effusion ... 176
Cardiac calcifications ... 177
Enlarged ascending aorta ... 179
Enlarged pulmonary arteries ... 180
Enlarged superior vena cava ... 182

## PERITONEUM, MESENTERY, AND RETROPERITONEUM ... 183
Pneumoperitoneum ... 184
Ascites ... 185
Abdominal abscess ... 187
Peritoneal lesion ... 189
Mesenteric mass ... 191
Retroperitoneal fibrosis ... 193
Retroperitoneal mass ... 194

## LIVER ... 197
Hepatomegaly ... 198
Low-density liver precontrast ... 202
Fatty liver ... 204
High-density liver precontrast ... 205

## CONTENTS

| | |
|---|---:|
| Hepatic calcifications | 206 |
| Liver lesion | 208 |
| Multiple liver lesions | 211 |
| Low-density liver lesion precontrast | 212 |
| Low-density liver lesion postcontrast | 215 |
| Liver cyst | 217 |
| Hypervascular liver lesion | 219 |
| Liver lesion with central scar | 221 |
| Portal venous gas | 222 |

**GALLBLADDER AND BILE DUCTS** — 223
- Enlarged gallbladder — 224
- Dilated common bile duct without obstruction — 225
- Intrahepatic biliary dilatation — 226
- Diffuse gallbladder-wall thickening — 228
- Focal gallbladder-wall thickening — 229
- High-altitude bile — 230
- Pneumobilia — 231

**SPLEEN** — 233
- Small spleen — 234
- Splenomegaly — 235
- Splenic lesion — 237
- Splenic cyst — 239
- Splenic calcifications — 240

**PANCREAS** — 241
- Pancreatic fatty change — 242
- Pancreatic calcification — 243
- Pancreatic cyst — 245
- Pancreatic mass — 246
- Hypervascular pancreatic mass — 249

**ADRENAL GLANDS** — 251
- Adrenal mass — 252
- Adrenal calcification — 254

**KIDNEYS** — 257
- Unilateral small kidney — 258
- Bilateral small kidneys — 259
- Unilateral large kidney — 260
- Bilateral large kidneys — 262
- Renal calcifications — 265
- Hydronephrosis — 268
- Renal mass — 269

## CONTENTS xi

   Renal mass with fat     273
   Renal cysts     274
   Perinephric lesion     277

**GASTROINTESTINAL TRACT**     279
   Dilated esophagus     280
   Narrowed esophagus     282
   Thickened or narrowed stomach     284
   Gastric mass     286
   Pneumatosis intestinalis     288
   Dilated small bowel     290
   Thickened small bowel     293
   Thickened terminal ileum     297
   Small bowel mass     299
   Enlarged, distended colon     301
   Colonic obstruction     302
   Thickened colon     303
   Colonic mass     306
   Narrowed cecum     308

**GENITOURINARY TRACT**     311
   Uretral dilatation     312
   Diffuse bladder-wall thickening     313
   Bladder calcification     314
   Filling defect in bladder     315
   Air in bladder wall or lumen     316
   Calcified seminal vesicles and VAS deferens     317
   Pelvic fluid     318
   Enlarged uterus     319
   Solid ovarian mass     321
   Cystic ovarian mass     324
   Calcified ovarian lesion     326

**CHEST AND ABDOMINAL WALL**     327
   Gynecomastia     328
   Body-wall mass     329
   Soft tissue calcifications     331
   Sclerotic bone lesion     333
   Lytic bone lesion     335
   Diffuse sclerosis     337

*Bibliography*     339
*Index*     345

# PREFACE

Modern CT techniques provide images with exquisite anatomic detail allowing detection and characterization of subtle disease processes. As a result, body CT has become a crucial component for diagnosis and management of a wide spectrum of medical and surgical conditions for both hospitalized and ambulatory patients. The wealth of information recorded on CT images provides radiologists with an extensive array of diagnostic information covering all organ systems.

The purpose of this book is to provide a concise yet complete resource detailing the potential disease processes associated with specific CT findings. We have provided this information in a format that lists items from most to least common within subcategories, i.e., neoplasm, inflammatory, congenital, etc. The most common entities are denoted by **boldface** type, and rare conditions or unusual manifestations of a disease are in *italicized* print. The right-hand column in each differential provides a summary of distinguishing morphologic characteristics and relevant clinical or pathologic details.

These lists have been developed from the information

available in the literature and classic textbooks (see Bibliography) balanced by our own clinical experience. We would like to thank the numerous faculty and residents at the Mallinckrodt Institute who offered suggestions and provided critical review of the contents as it evolved over the past year. We would like to give special thanks to Debra Brouk, Linda Macker, Mary Keller, and Anna Langenberg for their expert secretarial assistance; to Muza Navrozov, James Morgan, and Catherine Saggese at McGraw-Hill for their editorial efforts and important contributions in bringing this book to publication. It is our hope that this book provides a solid and helpful reference for your daily practice of radiology.

RMS
AJF

# ACRONYMS

| | |
|---|---|
| AAA | Abdominal aortic aneurysm |
| ABPA | Allergic bronchopulmonary aspergillosis |
| AI | Aortic insufficiency |
| AIDS | Acquired immune deficiency syndrome |
| AML | Acute myelogenous leukemia or angiomyolipoma |
| APCKD | Adult polycystic kidney disease |
| ARDS | Acute respiratory distress syndrome |
| AS | Aortic stenosis |
| ASD | Atrial septal defect |
| ATS | American Thoracic Society |
| AV | Atrioventricular |
| AVM | Arterial venous malformation |
| BAC | Bronchoalveolar cell carcinoma |
| BAL | Bronchoalveolar lavage |
| BCNU | Carmustine (chemotherapy) |
| BOOP | Bronchiolitis obliterans with organizing pneumonia |
| BPH | Benign prostatic hypertrophy |
| CAD | Coronary artery disease |

| | |
|---|---|
| CBD | Common bile duct |
| CHF | Congestive heart failure |
| CLL | Chronic lymphocytic leukemia |
| CML | Chronic myelogenous leukemia |
| CMV | Cytomegalovirus |
| CNS | Central nervous system |
| COPD | Chronic obstructive pulmonary disease |
| CPPD | Calcium pyrophosphate dihydrate deposition disease |
| CREST | *C*alcinosis of skin, *R*aynaud phenomenon, *E*sophageal dysmotility, *S*clerodactly, *T*elangiectasia |
| CT | Computed tomography |
| CVL | Central venous line |
| CXR | Chest x-ray |
| DIC | Disseminated intravascular coagulopathy |
| DIP | Desquamative interstitial pneumonitis |
| EG | Eosinophilic granuloma |
| ERCP | Endoscopic retrograde cholangiopancreatography |
| ESWL | Extracorporal shock wave lithotripsy |
| FD | Fibrous dysplasia |
| FMD | Fibromuscular dysplasia |
| GEJ | Gastroesophageal junction |
| HCC | Hepatocellular carcinoma |
| HIV | Human immunodeficiency virus |
| HRCT | High-resolution CT |
| HU | Hounsfield unit |
| IMA | Inferior mesenteric artery |
| IPF | Idiopathic pulmonary fibrosis |
| ITP | Idiopathic thrombocytopenic purpura |
| IVC | Inferior vena cava |

| | |
|---|---|
| LA | Left atrium |
| LLL | Left lower lobe |
| LUL | Left upper lobe |
| LV | Left ventricle |
| MAI | Mycobacterium avium intracellulare |
| MEN | Multiple endocrine neoplasia |
| MFH | Malignant fibrous histiocytoma |
| MI | Myocardial infarction |
| NF | Neurofibromatosis |
| NHL | Non-Hodgkin lymphoma |
| NSAID | Nonsteroidal anti-inflammatory drugs |
| PA | Pulmonary artery |
| PAPVR | Partial anomalous pulmonary venous return |
| PCP | *Pneumocystis carinii* pneumonia |
| PDA | Patent ductus arteriosus |
| PID | Pelvic inflammatory disease |
| PMF | Progressive massive fibrosis |
| PML | Polymorphonuclear leukocyte |
| PNET | Primitive neuroectodermal tumor |
| RA | Right atrium |
| RCCA | Renal cell carcinoma |
| RLQ | Right lower quadrant |
| ROI | Region of interest |
| RUQ | Right upper quadrant |
| RV | Right ventricle |
| SBO | Small bowel obstruction |
| SMA | Superior mesenteric artery |
| SMV | Superior mesenteric vein |
| STD | Sexually transmitted disease |
| SVC | Superior vena cava |
| TAPVR | Total anomalous pulmonary venous return |
| TCA | Tricyclic antidepressants |

| | |
|---|---|
| TE | Tracheoesophageal |
| THAD | Transient hepatic attenuation difference |
| TOA | Tuboovarian abscess |
| TS | Tuberous sclerosis |
| UIP | Usual interstitial pneumonitis |
| UPJ | Ureteropelvic junction |
| UVJ | Ureterovesicular junction |
| VHL | Von Hippel Lindau |
| VIP | Vasoactive intestinal peptide |
| VSD | Ventricular septal defect |

# FLEISHMAN'S 10 RULES OF BOARDMANSHIP

1. **TAKE control of each case.** Make the examiner **comfortable** with you as a consultant. Be confident but not cavalier or arrogant.
2. **BRIEFLY** identify the study. Be concise and don't perseverate, the idea is to help **orient yourself** to the study.
3. **BRIEFLY** describe the findings and don't beat them to death—PLEASE!!!
4. **MASTER** the anatomy, buzzwords, and imaging modality–specific lingo. These are the tools of your trade.
5. **PROVIDE** your own **history** by making hypothetical statements such as "If this patient had ____ symptom, it would suggest ____ disease."
6. **ASK** for contrast or the next study **when appropriate**. Be as specific as possible in your request and ask only after you have taken the initial images as far as you can. Ask only if it's going to have an impact on your differential. Be prepared to justify your request and to be denied.

7. **QUICKLY** offer a **limited differential diagnosis**. It is seldom necessary to mention more than three items. Always mention your **best diagnosis first. Never** mention something you know nothing about or an anecdotal case you've seen or heard about. **Don't** discuss at length an entity you know it's not.

8. **POLISH** your **best diagnosis** by taking it further if possible. Offer a relevant pathologic fact, clinical curiosity, or prognostic tidbit.

9. **ALWAYS** think about and discuss the **next appropriate imaging** step or other workup. Recommending this is your job as a radiologic consultant.

10. **ALWAYS** end with a **summary** to wrap the case up—don't silently wait for the examiner's move. Summarize the findings in a single phrase. State which diagnosis you favor most and why and recommend any further steps.

# ADENOPATHY

| Lymph nodes | Normal (short axis) |
| --- | --- |
| Submandibular (level I) | ≤ 1.1 cm * |
| High cervical (level II) | ≤ 1.1 cm * |
| Mid- and low cervical (levels III and IV) | ≤ 1.0 cm * |
| Spinal accessory (level V) | ≤ 1.0 cm * |
| Supraclavicular | ≤ 0.5 cm |
| Axillary | ≤ 1 cm, larger if center is fatty |
| High paratracheal and paraesophageal (ATS† levels 2, 8) | ≤8 mm |
| Low paratracheal and AP window (ATS levels 3, 4, 5) | ≤1.0 cm |
| Prevascular (ATS level 6) | ≤ 8 mm |
| Subcarinal (ATS level 7) | ≤ 12 mm |
| Hilar (ATS level 10) | ≤ 0.5 cm |
| Pericardial (ATS level 14) | ≤ 0.5 cm (no more than two) |
| Retrocrural | ≤ 6 mm |
| Gastrohepatic | ≤ 8 mm |
| Porta hepatis | ≤ 1.5 cm |
| Celiac axis | ≤ 1.0 cm |
| Retroperitoneal | ≤ 1.0 cm |
| Mesenteric | ≤ 1.0 cm |
| Pelvic | ≤ 1.0 cm |
| Inguinal | ≤ 1.0 cm |

In all cases, an increased number of lymph nodes despite normal size or a spherical shape, rather than ovoid, also suggests pathology.

* Regardless of size, central low density (not fat) is abnormal at any size. The majority of lymph nodes > 1.5 cm are malignant.

† ATS = American Thoracic Society.

# 1. CALCIFIED LYMPH NODES

| | |
|---|---|
| **Old granulomatous disease*** | Histoplasmosis, tuberculosis |
| **Silicosis** | May have "eggshell pattern," 2- to 5-mm upper lobe pulmonary nodules ± calcification, which may coalesce to PMF |
| Sarcoidosis | May have "eggshell pattern," variable pulmonary involvement ± adenopathy |
| *Disseminated pneumocystis carinii* | AIDS patients, bilateral perihilar interstitial or ground-glass pattern early; airspace, nodules, cysts, and pneumothorax when advanced |
| *Treated lymphoma* | Particularly Hodgkin |

* Here and in the following, common conditions are typeset in **bold**, rare in *italics*.

## 6 ADENOPATHY

| | |
|---|---|
| *Metastatic cancer* | Mucinous adenocarcinoma, osteosarcoma, medullary thyroid carcinoma |
| *Amyloidosis*\* | May be very dense, variable pulmonary appearance including interstitial disease and solitary or multiple nodules ± calcification or cavitation |

\* Here and in the following, common conditions are typeset in **bold**, rare in *italics*.

## 2. LOW-ATTENUATION ADENOPATHY

**Infection**  Pyogenic; fungal; mycobacterial, particularly tuberculosis; in the abdomen, ileocecal thickening often seen with tuberculosis or proximal small bowel thickening with MAI; HIV patients

**Metastases**  Bronchogenic, testicular, ovarian cancer

Postradiation therapy or chemotherapy  Especially lymphoma

Mesenteric adenitis

Whipple disease  Abdominal adenopathy, thick folds, no dilatation, normal transit time

## ADENOPATHY

| | |
|---|---|
| *Lymphangioleio-myomatosis* | Uniformly distributed thin-walled pulmonary cysts in young women; pneumothorax and chylous effusion common; tuberous sclerosis can appear similar |

## 3. HYPERVASCULAR LYMPH NODES

| | |
|---|---|
| Metastases | Renal cell, melanoma, thyroid, Kaposi sarcoma (AIDS), paraganglioma, carcinoid |
| Castleman disease | Angiofollicular lymph node hyperplasia—benign, idiopathic lymph node enlargement, may compress adjacent structures, striking contrast enhancement ± calcification, hyaline-vascular and plasma cell types |
| Lymphoma | Can have moderate enhancement |
| HIV-related adenopathy | Benign but indistinguishable from Kaposi sarcoma and metastatic disease (may be associated with lymphoepithelial cysts in the parotid gland) |

# LOWER NECK AND TRACHEA

## 4. NECK MASS

**Abscess**
Tonsil, parotid, dental procedure, trauma; thick enhancing wall, adjacent inflammation

Air-filled mass
Laryngocele, tracheal diverticulum, Zenker diverticulum, lateral pharyngeal diverticulum

Vascular
Aneurysm, posttraumatic pseudoaneurysm, ectatic vessels, asymmetric jugular veins, thromboses, pterygoid venous plexus, AVMs

Prevertebral space
Anterior disk herniation; vertebral body osteophytes; osteomyelitis, abscess; vertebral body metastases—lung, breast, prostate, non-Hodgkin lymphoma, chordoma; hematoma—fracture

## Adenopathy

**Lymphoma** — Non-Hodgkin may involve extranodal lymphatic tissue such as Waldeyer's ring

**Metastases** — Squamous cell carcinoma, melanoma, thyroid carcinoma

**Reactive** — Suppurative from pyogenic infection; low-density center, mycobacterial—particularly tuberculosis (scrofula), with characteristic thick peripheral enhancement

Calcified — Medullary thyroid cancer

## Tumor

**Malignant** — Squamous cell carcinoma—infiltrating mass

Benign — Parathyroid adenoma—usually adjacent and posterior to thyroid but may be ectopic
Hemangioma—enhancing mass, capillary and cavernous types
Pleomorphic adenoma—arises from minor or ectopic salivary gland

| | |
|---|---|
| | Lipoma—characteristic fat density
Others: benign mixed tumor, liposarcoma—very rare in neck, dermoid, angiofibroma |
| Neurogenic | Schwannoma (neurolemmoma)—fusiform mass along cranial nerves, may have cystic degeneration
Neurofibroma—low-density mass adjacent to carotid or in posterior cervical space
Plexiform neurofibroma—diffusely infiltrating and poorly circumscribed variant
Paraganglioma—carotid body tumors or glomus vagale, intense enhancement, 5% bilateral |

## 5. CYSTIC NECK MASS

**Necrotic adenopathy** — Particularly tonsillar and nasopharyngeal malignancies, thick irregular wall

**Abscess** — Pharyngitis, dental procedure, parotid, trauma; thick enhancing wall, adjacent inflammation

First branchial cleft cyst — Residual embryonic tract begins near submandibular triangle and ascends near parotid gland

Second branchial cleft cyst — Incomplete obliteration of branchial cleft tract, young to middle-aged adults, anterior triangle

Cervical thymic cyst — Forms along migratory tract of thymic tissue into the mediastinum

Thyroglossal duct cyst — Midline

Neurogenic cyst — Schwannoma—large lesions may undergo cystic degeneration, neurofibroma—low-density precontrast

## LOWER NECK AND TRACHEA

| | |
|---|---|
| Dermoid | Cystic teratoma (epidermoid, dermoid, or teratoid cyst) or nonteratomatous epithelium-lined cyst |
| Lymphangioma | Cystic hygroma—multilocular, thin-walled cystic mass, posterior triangle, more common in children |
| Miscellaneous | Thornwaldt cyst—nasopharyngeal roof, parathyroid cyst—adults in third and fourth decades, mucus-retention cyst, hemangioma, ranula, jugular venous thrombosis, bronchogenic cyst |

## 6. THORACIC INLET OR SUPERIOR MEDIASTINAL MASS

| | |
|---|---|
| **Thyroid mass** | Goiter, adenoma, carcinoma; may compress trachea or esophagus |
| **Lymphoma** or leukemia | Particularly CLL and Hodgkin disease |
| Adenopathy | Reactive; head and neck, bronchogenic and breast cancer |
| Tortuous brachiocephalic vessels | Elongate and become ectatic with age, atherosclerotic calcification common |
| Thymic mass | Thymoma, thymolipoma, thymic carcinoma, rebound hyperplasia, thymic cyst |
| Parathyroid mass | Adenoma |
| Cervical aorta | Very high aortic arch |
| Lymphangioma | Cystic hygroma—multilocular, thin-walled cystic mass, more common in children |

## 7. THYROID LESION

**Goiter** — Well-defined mass, often with cystic areas and calcification, large mass may extend into mediastinum

**Adenoma** — Adenomatous hyperplasia, follicular adenoma, ± calcification; parathyroid adenoma

Thyroid carcinoma — 50% have microcalcifications (psammoma bodies); papillary (>50%), follicular, anaplastic, medullary—associated with MEN 2 and 3, Hürthle cell; metastasizes to lung and bone

Cystic lesion — 20% of thyroid nodules; colloid cyst; colloid-filled macrofollicle in a goiter; simple cyst; necrotic papillary cancer, adenoma, or goiter; cystic parathyroid tumor

Inflammation — Thyroiditis, abscess

Hemorrhage — Within an adenoma or colloid nodule

| | |
|---|---|
| *Lymphoma* | Particularly Hodgkin |
| *Metastases* | Breast, lung, renal cell, melanoma |

## 8. ENLARGED PAROTID GLAND

| | |
|---|---|
| **Inflammatory** | Acute or chronic sialadenitis, sarcoidosis, mumps, tuberculosis, cat-scratch fever, actinomycosis, Sjögren disease |
| **Benign tumors** | Pleomorphic adenoma (>50%), papillary cystadenoma lymphomatosum (Warthin's tumor), oncocytoma, lymphangioma—thin-walled multilocular, lipoma, hemangioma—most common parotid tumor in child |
| Sialosis | Bilateral enlargement, metabolic disorders, drug reaction |
| Abscess | Thick, enhancing wall with low-density necrotic center |
| Malignant tumor | Mucoepidermoid, adenocarcinoma, adenoid cystic (cylindroma), lymphoma, acinic cell |

| | |
|---|---|
| Cyst | Lymphoepithelial cyst (AIDS patients), first branchial cleft cyst |
| Metastases | Squamous cell carcinoma, melanoma, non-Hodgkin lymphoma |
| Lymphoproliferative disease | Immunocompromised organ transplant recipients |

## 9. NARROWED LARYNX (true cords or subglottic)

| | |
|---|---|
| **Tumor** | Squamous cell carcinoma; benign—hemangioma, polyp, adenoma, fibroma, papilloma (most common mass in children) |
| **Inflammation** | Croup (subglottic inflammation), epiglottitis, tuberculosis, Wegener granulomatosis, sarcoidosis |
| **Vocal cord paralysis** | Birth injury, Chiari malformations, intracranial tumor, mediastinal mass or cyst, vascular ring, thyroidectomy or laryngeal malignancy |
| Congenital | Laryngeal atresia, stenosis, or web |
| Trauma | Foreign body, hematoma, prolonged endotracheal intubation |

# 10. TRACHEAL NARROWING

## Extrinsic

| | |
|---|---|
| **Mediastinal mass** | Thyroid mass (goiter); adenopathy—sarcoidosis, granulomatous disease, lymphoma, metastases (renal, lung, testicular); esophageal cancer; bronchogenic cyst |
| Central bronchogenic cancer | Particularly small cell, squamous cell |
| Fibrosis | Radiation, fibrosing mediastinitis—calcified adenopathy from histoplasmosis or tuberculosis |
| Saber-sheath trachea | Narrow width, advanced emphysema |
| *Vascular ring* | Right aortic arch with aberrant left subclavian, double aortic arch |

## Intrinsic

| | |
|---|---|
| **Trauma** | Burn or chemical aspiration |

| | |
|---|---|
| Cartilage deficiency | Tracheomalacia, prior tracheostomy, trauma, radiation therapy, intubation injury, congenital |
| Inflammation | Croup, tuberculosis, fungus, epidermolysis bullosa |
| Carcinoma | Squamous cell, adenoid cystic |

## With thickening

| | |
|---|---|
| Wegener granulomatosis | Idiopathic vasculitis involving upper and lower respiratory tract, arteries and veins, glomerulonephritis, pulmonary nodules ± cavitation |
| Sarcoidosis | Variable pulmonary involvement ± adenopathy, characteristic peribronchovascular nodules on HRCT |
| *Infection* | Tuberculosis, *Klebsiella* rhinoscleroma |

| | |
|---|---|
| *Relapsing polychondritis* | Idiopathic recurrent inflammation of cartilage (nose, ear, tracheobronchial tree) |
| *Tracheopathia osteoplastica* | Idiopathic disease characterized by cartilaginous nodules in the submucosa of the airway |
| *Amyloidosis* | Variable pulmonary involvement including interstitial disease and nodules $\pm$ calcification or cavitation |

## 11. TRACHEAL ENLARGEMENT
(> 26 mm in men and > 23 mm in women)

| | |
|---|---|
| **Tracheomalacia** | Endotracheal cuff damage |
| **Adjacent pulmonary fibrosis** | Particularly following radiation therapy |
| **Cystic fibrosis** | Autosomal recessive, hyperinflation, upper lobe–predominant peribronchial thickening, mucus plugging, progressive bronchiectasis, variable adenopathy |
| Tracheobronchomegaly | Mounier-Kuhn syndrome |
| Relapsing polychondritis | Idiopathic recurrent inflammation of cartilage (nose, ear, tracheobronchial tree) |
| *Uncommon* | Immunoglobulin deficiency, tracheocele; Ehlers-Danlos complex—rare systemic connective tissue disease, can cause tracheomegaly and bronchiectasis |

## 12. TRACHEAL OR ENDOBRONCHIAL MASS

### Tumors

| | |
|---|---|
| **Bronchogenic carcinoma** | Squamous cell—most common adenocarcinoma |
| **Adenoid cystic carcinoma** | Also called "cylindroma"; 25% of primary tracheal malignancies, smooth or polypoid, submucosal extension common |
| **Direct invasion** | Esophageal, lung, thyroid cancer |
| Carcinoid | Smooth, sharply marginated |
| Mucoepidermoid carcinoma | Salivary gland type of malignancy |
| Pleomorphic adenoma | |
| Benign tumor | Hemangioma, chondroma, fibroma, papilloma—most common laryngeal tumor in child, "drop metastases" in lung |

| | |
|---|---|
| *Endobronchial metastasis* | Renal cell, breast, melanoma, colon, lymphoma |
| **Other** | |
| **Mucus** | Asthma, allergic bronchopulmonary aspergillosis, congenital bronchial atresia |
| Foreign body | May be radiolucent, causes hyperinflation in child |
| *Broncholith* | Compression or erosion of a hilar lymph node into adjacent bronchus |

# LUNG

# GLOBAL PULMONARY PATTERNS

## 13. DIFFUSE LUNG DISEASE

### Pulmonary edema

| | |
|---|---|
| **Congestive heart failure** | Diffuse perihilar, lower lobe, and dependent pulmonary infiltrates, cardiomegaly, central vascular enlargement, pleural effusions common; MI, cardiomyopathy |
| **Fluid overload** | Hypervolemia; enlarged central vessels, thickened fissures, effusions |
| **Renal failure** | Cardiomegaly and central vascular enlargement, uremia |
| Valvular heart disease | Aortic stenosis, mitral stenosis |
| Noncardiogenic edema—ARDS | Pulmonary or systemic injury, cardiomegaly and effusions absent; trauma, burns, shock, sepsis, aspiration, pancreatitis, pneumonia, near-drowning, oxygen toxicity, |

|  |  |
|---|---|
|  | amniotic fluid or fat embolization; DIC; multiple transfusions; drug reaction—morphine, heroin, cocaine, aspirin, TCA; sickle cell; tumor; stroke or neurologic insult; toxic inhalation—hydrocarbon, nitrogen dioxide, sulfur dioxide, phosgene, carbon monoxide |
| *Uncommon causes* | Hypoproteinemia; lymphatic obstruction; high altitude; eclampsia; radiation pneumonitis; anaphylaxis; contrast reaction; upper airway obstruction; reexpansion edema; obstruction to venous return—pulmonary vein thrombosis, venoocclusive disease, fibrosing mediastinitis, left atrial thrombosis or myxoma |

## Pneumonia

| | |
|---|---|
| **Gram-positive bacteria** | Consolidation; *pneumococcus; S. aureus; actinomyces* and |

| | |
|---|---|
| | *Nocardia*—previously classified as fungus |
| **Gram-negative bacteria** | *Klebsiella; Pseudomonas*—hematogenous spread; *Legionella; H. influenzae; E. coli* |
| **Mycoplasma** | Interstitial pattern is most common |
| Anaerobic bacteria | Oral flora—*Bacteroides, Fusobacterium, Peptococcus* |
| Mycobacteria | Tuberculosis, *Mycobacterium avium-intracellulare* complex (MAI, MAC), *M. kansasii* |
| Fungus | Histoplasmosis, blastomycosis, aspergillosis, coccidiomycosis, cryptococcosis, candidiasis, mucormycosis |
| Viral | Interstitial pattern most common; mononucleosis, varicella—skin rash present, CMV |
| *Parasites* | Amebiasis, ascariasis, paragonimiasis |

## Opportunistic infections

| | |
|---|---|
| **Bacteria** | Pyogenic—*S. aureus, Pseudomonas; Legionella, Nocardia* |
| *Pneumocystis carinii* | Common pulmonary infection in AIDS; perihilar interstitial or ground-glass-opacities; airspace, nodules, cysts and pneumothorax when advanced; effusion and adenopathy rare; BAL usually diagnostic |
| Virus | CMV—common in transplant patients, interstitial pattern most common; varicella zoster, herpes |
| Mycobacteria | Particularly tuberculosis—patterns include primary, reactivation, or miliary, dependent on severity of immunosuppression; MAI |
| Fungus | Most commonly *Aspergillus* or *Candida,* also *Cryptococcus* and mucormycosis |
| *Parasites* | Toxoplasmosis, cryptosporidiosis, and |

strongyloidiasis occur as extrapulmonary infections in AIDS patients and rarely involve lung; patterns are variable

## Tumors

Broncho-alveolar cell carcinoma
: Can present as focal or multifocal consolidation, nodules, or a mass

Lymphangitic carcinomatosis
: Reticulonodular interstitial pattern ± peribronchovascular and subpleural thickening and effusion; breast and lung most common; also stomach, pancreas, and leukemia

Pulmonary metastases
: Smooth, round nodules of various sizes; lower lobe and peripheral predominance; hemorrhagic nodules may be ill-defined; squamous cell may cavitate

*Lymphoma*
: Usually non-Hodgkin; uncommon without adenopathy; nodules ± air bronchograms

## Other

Pulmonary fibrosis
Septal thickening, architectural distortion, cystic airspaces, ground-glass opacities, traction bronchiectasis, reduced lung volumes; idiopathic, drug-related, connective tissue disease, asbestosis, recurrent pneumonia, radiation therapy

Sarcoidosis
Variable pulmonary involvement ± adenopathy, interstitial thickening, ill-defined nodules and occasional alveolar pattern; peribronchovascular nodules on HRCT

Pulmonary hemorrhage
Focal or diffuse; bronchitis; bronchiectasis; pulmonary embolism; carcinoma; contusion; vasculitis—Goodpasture, lupus, Wegener; aspergilloma; anticoagulation; bleeding diathesis; AVM; DIC; vascular metastases; idiopathic

| | |
|---|---|
| Bronchiectasis | Enlarged, thickened bronchi from chronic inflammation; cylindrical, varicose, and cystic patterns; diffuse from cystic fibrosis or immotile cilia syndrome; central in ABPA |
| Hypersensitivity pneumonitis | Immunologic response to inhaled organic antigens; bilateral small nodules, ground-glass opacities and septal lines; fibrosis with chronic exposure |
| Eosinophilic granuloma | Upper lobe–predominant interstitial disease with preserved lung volumes, a variable combination of small nodules and cysts, fibrosis and pneumothorax may develop |
| *Silicosis and coal worker's pneumoconiosis* | Small upper lobe–predominant, frequently calcified nodules and septal thickening, may coalesce to PMF, calcified nodes common; stannosis, berylliosis, and siderosis are similar |

## DIFFUSE LUNG DISEASE

*Alveolar proteinosis*
Idiopathic overproduction (or decreased resorption) of surfactant by pneumocytes; diffuse, symmetric airspace disease with septal thickening "crazy paving" CT pattern is characteristic; treatment with BAL; predisposed to infection, particularly *Nocardia*

*Lymphangio-leiomyomatosis*
Uniformly distributed thin-walled pulmonary cysts and preserved or increased lung volumes in young women; pneumothorax and chylous effusion common complicating features; tuberous sclerosis can appear similar

## 14. DIFFUSE INTERSTITIAL LUNG DISEASE WITH NORMAL OR INCREASED LUNG VOLUMES

**Emphysema**  Superimposed on diffuse disease of another cause

**Cystic fibrosis**  Autosomal recessive; hyperinflation, upper lobe–predominant bronchiectasis and variable adenopathy; sinus disease and pancreatic insufficiency

Eosinophilic granuloma  Upper lobe–predominant interstitial disease with a variable combination of small nodules and cysts; fibrosis and pneumothorax may develop

*Lymphangio-leiomyomatosis*  Uniformly distributed thin-walled pulmonary cysts in young women; pneumothorax and chylous effusion common complications; tuberous sclerosis can appear similar

## 15. PERIPHERAL LUNG DISEASE

**Pulmonary fibrosis**
Coarse septal interstitial thickening with architectural distortion, cystic airspaces, ground-glass opacities, and traction bronchiectasis
Idiopathic—IPF, DIP, UIP
Asbestosis—almost always concomitant pleural plaques
Drugs—bleomycin, BCNU, amiodarone, nitrofurantoin, methysergide, procainamide, busulfan, cyclophosphamide, methotrexate
Connective tissue disease—scleroderma (thickened soft tissues, esophageal dysmotility), lupus (pleural and pericardial effusions), rheumatoid, dermatomyositis
Recurrent pneumonia—often associated bronchiectasis

**Pneumonia**
Airspace disease—bacterial (aspiration), BOOP, eosinophilic

| | |
|---|---|
| Pulmonary metastases | Smooth, round nodules of various sizes; lower lobe and peripheral predominance; hemorrhagic nodules may be ill-defined |
| Sarcoidosis | Widely variable pulmonary patterns ± adenopathy including interstitial thickening, ill-defined nodules, and occasional alveolar pattern; peribronchovascular nodules on HRCT |
| *Hypersensitivity pneumonitis* | Immunologic response to inhaled organic antigens; bilateral small nodules, ground-glass opacities and septal lines; chronic exposure leads to fibrosis |
| *Pulmonary edema* | CHF, fluid overload, renal failure |
| *Pulmonary infarction* | |

## 16. PERIHILAR LUNG DISEASE

| | |
|---|---|
| **Pulmonary edema** | CHF, valvular heart disease, renal failure, fluid overload |
| Bronchitis | Bronchial wall thickening but no dilatation |
| Viral pneumonia | Generally symmetric, perihilar interstitial infiltrate |
| *Pneumocystis carinii* pneumonia | Common infection in AIDS; perihilar interstitial or ground-glass opacities; airspace, nodules, cysts, and pneumothorax when advanced; effusion and adenopathy rare |
| Sarcoidosis | Variable pulmonary patterns ± adenopathy including interstitial thickening and ill-defined nodules, peribronchovascular nodules on HRCT |

| | |
|---|---|
| Allergic bronchopulmonary aspergillosis | Central cylindrical bronchiectasis and mucus plugging colonized with *Aspergillus* in patients with asthma |
| *Alveolar proteinosis* | Idiopathic overproduction (or decreased resorption) of surfactant by pneumocytes; diffuse, symmetric airspace disease with septal thickening "crazy paving" CT pattern is characteristic; treatment with BAL; predisposed to infection, particularly *Nocardia* |

## 17. UPPER LUNG DISEASE

**Active granulomatous disease**
Post–primary tuberculosis (consolidation, nodules, cavitation), histoplasmosis

**Fibrosis**
Prior granulomatous disease, tuberculosis or histoplasmosis most commonly; radiation therapy to neck, shoulder, upper lobes or superior mediastinum

Cystic fibrosis
Hyperinflation, upper lobe–predominant bronchiectasis and mucus plugging, variable adenopathy

Sarcoidosis
Widely variable pulmonary patterns including nodules, interstitial and airspace disease, fibrosis in stage IV disease, may spare apex and base

Eosinophilic granuloma
Upper lobe–predominant interstitial disease with variable combination of small nodules or cysts; fibrosis and pneumothorax may develop

| | |
|---|---|
| Silicosis and coal worker's pneumoconiosis | Small upper lobe–predominant, frequently calcified nodules and septal thickening, may coalesce to PMF, calcified nodes common; stannosis, berylliosis, and siderosis are similar |
| *Ankylosing spondylitis* | Apical fibrosis, symmetric syndesmophytes, spinal and SI joint fusion |
| *Pulmonary edema* | Neurogenic, high altitude |

## 18. LOWER LUNG DISEASE

**Pneumonia**  Bacterial—consolidation with air bronchograms; aspiration—recurrent pneumonia from anaerobes and gram-negative organisms leads to lower lobe and posterior segment fibrosis; alcoholism; debilitation; neurologic disorder; esophageal disease; TE fistula; lipoid from chronic oil aspiration

**Atelectasis**  Immobilization, splinting from abdominal or chest pain, associated with effusions

**Pulmonary fibrosis**  Nodular thickening with architectural distortion, cystic airspaces, and traction bronchiectasis
Idiopathic (IPF)—DIP, UIP
Drugs—bleomycin, amiodarone, nitrofurantoin, BCNU, methysergide, procainamide,

| | |
|---|---|
| | busulfan, cyclophosphamide, methotrexate<br>Asbestosis—often see concomitant pleural plaques<br>Connective tissue disease—scleroderma (thickened soft tissues, esophageal dysmotility), lupus (small pleural and pericardial effusions), rheumatoid lung, dermatomyositis<br>Chronic pneumonia—often associated bronchiectasis |
| Pulmonary metastases | Smooth, round nodules of various sizes; lower lobe and peripheral predominance; hemorrhagic nodules may be ill-defined |
| Kaposi sarcoma | Almost exclusively AIDS-related; rare without preceding cutaneous involvement; typically bilateral nodular peribronchovascular process |

| | |
|---|---|
| *Acute hypersensitivity pneumonitis* | Immunologic response to inhaled organic antigens; diffuse small nodules, ground-glass opacities and septal lines that resolve over weeks |
| *Neuro-fibromatosis* | Lung involvement in about 20%; basilar bullae and interstitial thickening progressing to fibrosis |

## 19. HYPERLUCENT LUNG

| | |
|---|---|
| **Emphysema** | Hyperinflation, oligemia |
| **Compensatory hyperinflation** | Lobectomy or lobar collapse |
| Cystic fibrosis | Hyperinflation with upper lobe–predominant bronchiectasis and mucus plugging |
| Pulmonary hypertension | Central pulmonary artery enlargement |
| *Congenital heart disease* | Right-to-left shunt |
| *Bronchiolitis obliterans* | Small airway inflammation; ground-glass opacities, small centrilobular nodules, and "tree-in-bud" opacities on HRCT; air trapping on expiration |

## Unilateral

| | |
|---|---|
| Endobronchial obstruction* | One-way valve effect due to mucus plug, bronchogenic carcinoma, broncholith, carcinoid, foreign body, endobronchial metastasis |
| *Decreased vascularity* | Pulmonary thromboembolism, pulmonary artery hypoplasia or agenesis, hypogenetic lung—scimitar syndrome, congenital lobar emphysema; Swyer-James-MacLeod syndrome—unilateral oligemia from bronchiolitis obliterans in childhood |
| *Congenital bronchial atresia* | Blind-ending bronchus with mucus plug and peripheral oligemia; LUL most commonly |

* Postobstructive air trapping may be seen in child; collapse more common in adult.

## 20. ASYMMETRIC LUNG SIZE

**Pulmonary collapse** — Obstruction with foreign body, endobronchial tumor, or mucus

**Prior partial pulmonary resection** — Thoracotomy; displaced fissure, surgical staples along fissure or bronchus

**Phrenic nerve paralysis** — Surgery, tumor, idiopathic

**Eventration of hemidiaphragm** — Broad-based, most commonly right anterior portion

Abdominal displacement of hemidiaphragm — Distended stomach or colon, enlarged liver or spleen, subphrenic mass or fluid collection

*Uncommon causes* — Hypoplastic lung, asymmetric emphysema, unilateral lung transplant, diaphragmatic hernia, congenital lobar emphysema, fibrothorax, mesothelioma, thoracoplasty

## 21. ATELECTASIS AND PULMONARY COLLAPSE

| | |
|---|---|
| **Obstructive** | Endobronchial lesion—bronchogenic carcinoma, mucus plug, carcinoid, foreign body, broncholith, endobronchial metastasis, benign stricture |
| **Passive** | Pleural effusion, pleural mass, pneumothorax, scoliosis |
| Cicatrizing (scar) | Fibrosis; granulomatous disease—tuberculosis, histoplasmosis; connective tissue—scleroderma, lupus, rheumatoid; IPF; radiation therapy; sarcoidosis |
| Compressive | Parenchymal tumor, bullous emphysema |
| *Adhesive* | Respiratory distress syndrome, pulmonary embolism |

## 22. BRONCHIECTASIS*

| | |
|---|---|
| **Recurrent pneumonia** | Particularly childhood infections; aspiration, obstructing tumor |
| **Fibrosis— traction bronchiectasis** | Radiation therapy, infection, IPF, connective tissue disease, sarcoidosis |
| Congenital | Cystic fibrosis—predominantly upper lobe cystic and cylindrical, hyperinflation and mucus plugging<br>Cartilage deficiency<br>Immune deficiency—agammaglobulinemia<br>Immotile cilia syndrome—Kartagener syndrome |
| *ABPA* | Central bronchiectasis, patients with asthma |
| Artifact | Respiratory or cardiac motion |
| *Tracheobronchomegaly* | Mounier-Kuhn syndrome—central bronchiectasis |

* Bronchiectasis may be transient following pneumonia in children.

| | |
|---|---|
| *Poststenotic* | Endobronchial lesion or extrinsic compression |
| *Inhalation injury* | Toxic fumes, smoke, chemicals |

# PULMONARY CYSTS AND NODULES

## 23. SOLITARY PULMONARY NODULE* (< 3 cm)

### Inflammatory

| | |
|---|---|
| **Granuloma** | Usually small, smooth, often calcified when healed; tuberculosis, histoplasmosis, coccidiomycosis |
| **Scar** | Postinflammatory, often linear and extending to pleura |
| **Round pneumonia** | Round area of consolidation with ill-defined borders and air bronchograms; almost exclusively in children; *Pneumococcus, Legionella, Nocardia, Streptococcus* |
| Aspergilloma | In preexisting cavity |
| Organizing pneumonia | Bacterial—*Nocardia, Actinomyces;* air bronchograms, may be associated with bronchiolitis obliterans |

* Rarely malignant before age 40.

| | |
|---|---|
| Lung abscess | Circular, thick, irregular walls, may be fluid-filled and appear solid; bacterial most common, amebic |
| Fungus | Particularly immunocompromised patient; aspergillosis, blastomycosis, coccidiomycosis, cryptococcosis, histoplasmosis |
| *Rheumatoid* | Necrobiotic nodule—often multiple and may cavitate |
| *Echinococcal cyst* | Hydatid disease; round cystic mass, ± air/fluid level, water lily sign |

## Neoplasms

| | |
|---|---|
| **Bronchogenic carcinoma** | Irregular or spiculated mass; adenocarcinoma (bronchoalveolar), squamous, large cell; often metastatic at presentation |

| | |
|---|---|
| **Metastasis** | Usually multiple; breast, sarcoma, colon, melanoma, renal cell, testicular |
| **Hamartoma** | Most common benign neoplasm, smooth or lobulated; 30% calcify, 50% contain fat |
| Carcinoid | 80% are central |
| Pseudotumor | Loculated fluid in fissure |
| *Pleural tumor* | Fibrous tumor—visceral pleural attachment in fissure may simulate pulmonary nodule |
| *Lymphoma* | Non-Hodgkin; more common with recurrence, usually adenopathy; mass ± air bronchograms |

## Vascular

| | |
|---|---|
| Wegener granulomatosis | Idiopathic vasculitis involving respiratory tract, arteries, and veins; glomerulonephritis; pulmonary nodules or focal consolidation ± cavitation |

## SOLITARY PULMONARY NODULE 57

| | |
|---|---|
| Pulmonary infarct | Pleural-based, wedge-shaped; may see areas of mosaic perfusion, intravascular emboli, volume loss, or effusion |
| Arteriovenous malformation | Well-defined lobular lesions feeding artery and draining vein, often associated with Osler-Weber-Rendu, increased risk of cerebral abscess |
| Hematoma | Evidence of trauma, resolves over weeks |
| *PA pseudoaneurysm* | Caused by overinflated pulmonary artery catheter |
| *Pulmonary vein varix* | Focal dilatation of pulmonary vein, typically near LA |

### Other causes

| | |
|---|---|
| **Rounded atelectasis** | Adjacent pleural disease, vessels and bronchi classically seen spiraling into mass |
| Lymph node | Benign intrapulmonary, peripheral, usually oval, 2 to 4 mm |

| | |
|---|---|
| Bronchogenic cyst | 15% are intrapulmonary, sharply marginated fluid-filled mass, usually near carina |
| Bronchocele/ mucoid impaction | Bronchiectasis; ABPA—asthmatics, central bronchiectasis with mucus plugs colonized by *Aspergillus;* bronchial atresia—congenital blind-ending bronchus with mucus plug and peripheral oligemia; bronchiectasis, cystic fibrosis |
| *Amyloidosis* | Interstitial disease and nodules ± calcification or cavitation |

## 24. SOLITARY PULMONARY MASS (>3 cm)

### Tumors

| | |
|---|---|
| **Bronchogenic cancer** | Irregular or spiculated mass; adenocarcinoma, squamous, large cell, BAC; often metastatic at presentation |
| Solitary metastasis | Breast, sarcoma, colon, melanoma, renal cell, testicular |
| Pseudotumor | Loculated fluid in fissure |
| Hamartoma | Most common benign neoplasm, smooth or lobulated; 30% calcify, 50% contain fat |
| *Pleural tumor* | Fibrous tumor—visceral pleural attachment in fissure may simulate pulmonary mass |
| *Lymphoma* | Non-Hodgkin; more common with recurrence, usually adenopathy; nodules ± air bronchograms |

## Inflammatory

| | |
|---|---|
| **Organized pneumonia** | Bacterial—*Nocardia, Actinomyces;* air bronchograms, may be associated with bronchiolitis obliterans |
| **Lung abscess** | Circular, thick, irregular walls, may be fluid-filled and appear solid; bacterial most common, amebic |
| **Round pneumonia** | Round area of consolidation with ill-defined borders and air bronchograms; almost exclusively in children; *Pneumococcus, Legionella, Nocardia, Streptococcus* |
| Granuloma | Usually small, smooth, often calcified; tuberculosis—satellite lesions common, histoplasmosis, coccidiomycosis |
| Fungus (active) | Particularly immunocompromised patient; aspergillosis, blastomycosis, coccidiomycosis, |

| | |
|---|---|
| | cryptococcosis, histoplasmosis |
| *Echinococcal cyst* | Hydatid disease; round, cystic mass, water lily sign |
| *Lipoid pneumonia* | Chronic oil aspiration, areas of fat density |

## Other

| | |
|---|---|
| **Rounded atelectasis** | Adjacent pleural disease, vessels and bronchi classically seen spiraling into mass |
| Bronchogenic cyst | 15% are intrapulmonary; sharply marginated fluid-filled mass, usually near carina |
| Hematoma | Evidence of trauma, mass resolves over weeks |
| Progressive massive fibrosis | Usually bilateral and asymmetric masses representing conglomeration of smaller nodules from silicosis or coal worker's pneumoconiosis; traction bronchiectasis common; may cavitate |

| | |
|---|---|
| Wegener granulomatosis | Idiopathic vasculitis involving respiratory tract, arteries, and veins; glomerulonephritis; pulmonary nodules or focal consolidation ± cavitation |
| *Pulmonary sequestration* | Congenital malformation with systemic arterial supply; LLL most common |
| *Cystic adenomatoid malformation* | Cystic and solid varieties, fluid-filled at birth, often associated lobar enlargement |

## 25. PERIPHERAL PULMONARY MASS

| | |
|---|---|
| **Bronchogenic carcinoma** | Most commonly adenocarcinoma or large cell |
| **Rounded atelectasis** | Adjacent pleural disease, vessels and bronchi classically seen spiraling into mass |
| **Organized pneumonia** | Bacterial—*Nocardia, Actinomyces;* air bronchograms, may be associated with bronchiolitis obliterans (BOOP) |
| **Granuloma** | Usually small, smooth, often calcified when healed; tuberculosis, histoplasmosis, coccidiomycosis |
| Metastasis | Usually smooth, peripheral, and multiple |
| Pulmonary infarct | Pleural-based, wedge-shaped; may include mosaic perfusion, intravascular emboli, volume loss, or effusion |

| | |
|---|---|
| *Lymphoma* | Non-Hodgkin; more common with recurrence, usually adenopathy; mass ± air bronchograms |
| *Pleural tumor* | Mesothelioma—usually associated effusion; fibrous tumor |
| *Sequestration* | Congenital malformation with systemic arterial supply; LLL most common; extralobar—systemic venous drainage; intralobar—pulmonary venous drainage |

# 26. CAVITARY LUNG LESION

## Inflammatory

**Lung abscess or necrotizing pneumonia** — Thick irregular wall, often aspiration related; bacterial—*Staphylococcus, Pseudomonas, Klebsiella, E. coli,* gram-negative organisms, anaerobes, *Actinomyces, Nocardia;* fungal—blastomycosis, aspergillosis, histoplasmosis, coccidiomycosis, cryptococcosis, mucormycosis; amebic

*Mycobacterial* — Tuberculosis most common, upper lobe, associated scarring; may colonize with *Aspergillus*

*Rheumatoid* — Necrobiotic nodule—often multiple

*Echinococcal cyst* — Hydatid disease, round cystic mass

## Tumors

**Bronchogenic carcinoma** — Classically squamous cell, also adenocarcinoma, particularly bronchoalveolar

Metastasis — Usually multiple, smooth, and peripheral; 5% cavitate; usually squamous cell of head and neck or cervix, sarcoma

*Carcinoid tumor* — Low-grade malignant endobronchial tumor; can calcify

*Lymphoma* — Pulmonary involvement more common with non-Hodgkin, but Hodgkin more likely to cavitate

## Congenital

Bronchogenic cyst — 15% are intrapulmonary, sharply marginated fluid-filled mass usually near carina; infection can lead to bronchial communication and air-fluid level

Intrapulmonary sequestration — Systemic arterial supply; LLL most common

| | |
|---|---|
| *Cystic adenomatoid malformation* | Cystic and solid varieties, fluid-filled at birth, often associated lobar enlargement |

## Vascular

| | |
|---|---|
| Wegener granulomatosis | Idiopathic vasculitis involving respiratory tract, arteries, and veins; glomerulonephritis; multiple nodules or focal consolidation |
| Septic emboli | Multiple peripheral, ill-defined nodular opacities, may include vessel leading to lesion; air bronchograms common; endocarditis, septic thrombophlebitis, catheters, drug users; *S. aureus,* gram-negative, anaerobes, streptococcus |
| Pulmonary infarct | Pleural-based, wedge-shaped; may include mosaic perfusion, intravascular emboli, volume loss, or effusion |
| Hematoma | Trauma |

## Other causes

Progressive massive fibrosis
Usually bilateral masses representing conglomerate of smaller nodules from silicosis or coal worker's pneumoconiosis; traction bronchiectasis common

*Amyloidosis*
Interstitial disease and solitary or multiple nodules ± calcification or cavitation

## 27. MULTIPLE LUCENT LESIONS OR CYSTS

**Bullae and blebs**  Emphysema, blebs arise in visceral pleura and are ≤1 cm, bullae are intrapulmonary air cysts >1 cm

**Loculated pneumothorax**  Separation of visceral and parietal pleura

**Pneumatoceles**  Trauma—healed hematoma or laceration; infection—*S. aureus; H. influenzae;* gram-negative organisms; PCP; tuberculosis

**Bronchiectasis**  Enlarged, thickened bronchi from chronic inflammation; cylindrical, varicose, and cystic; focal often idiopathic; diffuse from cystic fibrosis or immotile cilia syndrome; central with ABPA

Fibrosis with honeycombing  Nodular thickening with architectural distortion, cystic airspaces and traction bronchiectasis; idiopathic; drugs; connective tissue

| | |
|---|---|
| | disease—scleroderma, lupus, rheumatoid; asbestosis; chronic pneumonia; sarcoidosis |
| Eosinophilic granuloma | Upper lobe–predominant interstitial disease with a variable combination of small nodules and cysts; fibrosis and pneumothorax may develop |
| Abscess cavity | Active usually have thick wall with adjacent consolidation, may heal with thin wall, tuberculosis |
| *Necrotic metastases* | Usually thick-walled and multiple |
| *Cystic adenomatoid malformation* | Congenital lesion with cystic and solid varieties, fluid-filled at birth, often associated lobar enlargement |
| *Congenital lobar emphysema* | Multiple cystic airspaces with associated lobar enlargement |

| | |
|---|---|
| *Sequestration* | Congenital malformation with systemic arterial supply; LLL most common |
| *Bronchogenic cyst* | 15% intrapulmonary, may be air-filled following infection and communicate with bronchus |
| *Tracheobronchial papillomatosis* | Multiple tracheal and endobronchial lesions; may cavitate or cause postobstructive pneumonia |
| *Lymphangio-leiomyomatosis* | Uniformly distributed thin-walled cysts in young women; pneumothorax and chylous effusion common complications; tuberous sclerosis appears similar |
| *Prior echinococcal cyst* | Hydatid disease; round cystic mass |

## 28. MULTIPLE WELL-DEFINED PULMONARY NODULES

**Granulomatous disease**
Mycobacterial—tuberculosis, MAI
Fungus—histoplasmosis, coccidiomycosis, cryptococcosis

**Tumors**

**Metastases**
Smooth, round nodules of various sizes; lower lobe and peripheral predominance; hemorrhagic nodules may be ill-defined; 5% cavitate; most often squamous cell or sarcoma
Large—sarcoma, seminoma, renal cell, thyroid, colon
Miliary—thyroid, lung, breast, melanoma, renal cell
Calcified—mucinous adenocarcinoma, osteosarcoma, chondrosarcoma
Most likely to metastasize—choriocarcinoma, melanoma, sarcoma, renal cell, thyroid,

| | breast, testicular<br>Most likely origin—breast, renal, head and neck, colon |
|---|---|
| Bronchoalveolar cell carcinoma | Type of adenocarcinoma, can present as focal or multifocal consolidation, nodules or a mass ± cavitation |
| *Papillomas* | Frequently cavitate |
| *Lymphoma* | Non-Hodgkin; more common with recurrence, usually adenopathy; nodules ± air bronchograms |

## Vascular

| | |
|---|---|
| **Wegener granulomatosis** | Idiopathic vasculitis involving upper and lower respiratory tract, arteries, and veins; glomerulonephritis; multiple pulmonary nodules or focal consolidation ± cavitation |
| Arteriovenous malformations | Well-defined lobular lesions, feeding artery and draining vein; half associated with Osler-Weber-Rendu |

| | |
|---|---|
| Pulmonary infarcts | Pleural-based, wedge-shaped; may include mosaic perfusion, intravascular emboli, volume loss, or effusion |

## Other causes

| | |
|---|---|
| Silicosis and coal worker's pneumoconiosis | Small upper lobe–predominant, frequently calcified nodules and septal thickening, may coalesce to PMF, calcified nodes common; stannosis, berylliosis, and siderosis are similar |
| Eosinophilic granuloma | Upper lobe–predominant interstitial disease with a variable combination of small nodules and cysts; fibrosis and pneumothorax may develop |
| Mucoid impaction | Particularly allergic bronchopulmonary aspergillosis |
| *Sarcoidosis* | Variable pulmonary pattern ± adenopathy including nodules; tiny |

|   |   |
|---|---|
|  | peribronchovascular nodules on HRCT |
| *Amyloidosis* | Interstitial disease and nodules ± calcification or cavitation |
| *Rheumatoid* | Necrobiotic nodules—often multiple and can cavitate |

## 29. MULTIPLE ILL-DEFINED PULMONARY NODULES

### Infection

| | |
|---|---|
| **Granulomatous disease** | Tuberculosis, histoplasmosis, coccidiomycosis, cryptococcosis; often heal with calcification |
| Bacterial | Organizing bronchopneumonia, *Nocardia, Actinomyces, Legionella* |

### Tumors

| | |
|---|---|
| **Metastases** | Renal cell, thyroid, choriocarcinoma, colon, hemorrhagic—melanoma |
| Bronchoalveolar cell carcinoma | Variable patterns including focal or multifocal consolidation, nodules, or mass |
| Kaposi sarcoma | Almost exclusively AIDS-related; rare without preceding cutaneous involvement; typically lower |

lobe bilateral nodular peribronchovascular process

## Vascular

**Wegener granulomatosis** — Idiopathic vasculitis involving respiratory tract, arteries, and veins; glomerulonephritis; multiple pulmonary nodules or consolidation ± cavitation

**Septic emboli** — Multiple, peripheral, ill-defined nodular opacities, may include vessel leading to lesion; air bronchograms and cavitation common; endocarditis, septic thrombophlebitis, catheters, drug users; *S. aureus,* gram-negative, anaerobes, *Streptococcus*

Pulmonary infarcts — Pleural-based, wedge-shaped; mosaic perfusion, intravascular emboli, volume loss, or effusion

## Other causes

*Sarcoidosis*  Widely variable pulmonary patterns ± adenopathy including interstitial thickening and ill-defined nodules; peribronchovascular nodules on HRCT

Hypersensitivity pneumonitis  Immunologic response to inhaled organic antigens; small nodules, ground-glass appearance and septal lines that clear over weeks; chronic exposure leads to fibrosis

Eosinophilic granuloma  Upper lobe–predominant interstitial disease with a variable combination of small nodules and cysts; fibrosis and pneumothorax may develop

*Amyloidosis*  Interstitial disease and nodules ± calcification or cavitation

*Lymphoma*  Non-Hodgkin; more common with recurrence, usually adenopathy; ill-defined nodules ± air bronchograms

## 30. MULTIPLE CAVITARY NODULES

### Inflammatory

**Septic emboli**  Multiple peripheral, ill-defined nodular opacities, may include vessel leading to lesion; air bronchograms and cavitation common; endocarditis, septic thrombophlebitis, catheters, drug users; *S. aureus,* gram-negative, anaerobes, *Streptococcus*

Pneumonia  Fungus—particularly coccidioidomycosis; MAI and tuberculosis—nodular infiltrate

### Tumors

**Pulmonary metastases**  Smooth, round nodules of various sizes; lower lobe and peripheral predominance; 5% cavitate; most often squamous cell from head and neck, cervix, or sarcoma

Bronchoalveolar cell carcinoma  Uncommon pattern

| | |
|---|---|
| *Lymphoma* | Non-Hodgkin most common; pulmonary involvement more common late or with recurrence, usually mediastinal adenopathy; ill-defined solitary and multiple nodules ± air bronchograms |
| *Tracheobronchial papillomatosis* | Multiple tracheal and endobronchial lesions; may cavitate or cause postobstructive pneumonia |

## Other causes

| | |
|---|---|
| Eosinophilic granuloma | Upper lobe–predominant interstitial disease with a variable combination of small nodules and cysts; fibrosis and pneumothorax may develop |
| Progressive massive fibrosis (PMF) | Usually bilateral masses representing conglomeration of smaller nodules from silicosis or coal worker's pneumoconiosis; traction bronchiectasis common |
| Wegener granulomatosis | Idiopathic vasculitis involving respiratory tract, |

| | |
|---|---|
| | arteries, and veins; glomerulonephritis; multiple pulmonary nodules or focal consolidation ± cavitation |
| *Rheumatoid* | Necrobiotic nodules—often multiple and cavitate |
| *Multiple pulmonary infarcts* | Pleural-based, wedge-shaped; may include mosaic perfusion, intravascular emboli, volume loss, or effusion |
| *Amyloidosis* | Interstitial disease and nodules ± calcification or cavitation |

## 31. TINY NODULES (<5 mm; micronodular; miliary)

### Inflammatory

| | |
|---|---|
| **Granulomatous disease** | Histoplasmosis—calcification and frequently calcified lymph nodes; blastomycosis; coccidiomycosis |
| Miliary tuberculosis | Typically very ill or immunocompromised patient |
| Viral pneumonia | Particularly varicella—skin lesions invariably present |
| *Bacteria* | Particularly *Nocardia*—high-order bacteria |
| *Hypersensitivity pneumonitis* | Immunologic response to inhaled organic antigens; small nodules, ground-glass appearance |
| *Bronchiolitis obliterans; Asian panbronchiolitis* | Small airway inflammation; ground-glass attenuation, small centrilobular nodules and "tree-in-bud" opacities on HRCT; air trapping on expiration |

## Malignant

**Metastases** — Thyroid, melanoma, pancreas, renal, choriocarcinoma

Bronchoalveolar cell carcinoma — More often presents as focal or multifocal consolidation, nodules, or a mass

Lymphangitic carcinomatosis — Nodular interstitial process ± peribronchovascular and subpleural thickening and effusion; breast and lung most common, also stomach, pancreas, and leukemia

## Other causes

**Sarcoidosis** — Widely variable pulmonary patterns ± adenopathy including interstitial thickening and ill-defined nodules; peribronchovascular nodules on HRCT

**Silicosis and coal worker's pneumoconiosis** — Small upper lobe–predominant, frequently calcified nodules and septal thickening, may coalesce to PMF, calcified nodes common; siderosis,

|   |   |
|---|---|
|  | berylliosis, and stannosis are similar |
| Eosinophilic granuloma | Upper lobe–predominant interstitial disease with a variable combination of small nodules and cysts; fibrosis and pneumothorax may develop |
| *Alveolar microlithiasis* | Idiopathic with familial tendency; diffuse tiny (<1 mm) pulmonary calcifications |
| *Amyloidosis* | Interstitial disease and nodules ± calcification or cavitation |
| *Idiopathic pulmonary hemosiderosis* | Recurrent pulmonary hemorrhage leads to septal thickening and eventual fibrosis |

## 32. PULMONARY NODULES WITH ADENOPATHY

**Sarcoidosis** — Widely variable pulmonary patterns ± adenopathy including interstitial thickening and ill-defined nodules; characteristic peribronchovascular nodules on HRCT

**Metastatic disease** — Testicular, renal cell, lung

**Granulomatous infection** — Mycobacterial, particularly primary tuberculosis and fungal infections

Lymphoma — Usually non-Hodgkin; more common with recurrence, nodules ± air bronchograms

Silicosis and coal worker's pneumoconiosis — Small upper lobe–predominant, frequently calcified nodules and septal thickening, may coalesce to PMF and honeycombing, calcified nodes common; stannosis, berylliosis, and siderosis are similar

## 33. CALCIFIED PULMONARY NODULES

**Old healed granulomatous disease** — Histoplasmosis, coccidiomycosis, tuberculosis; frequently calcified lymph nodes

Hamartoma — 30% contain calcifications, 50% contain visible fat

Silicosis and coal worker's pneumoconiosis — Small upper lobe–predominant nodules which may coalesce to PMF, calcified nodes common

Varicella pneumonia — Healed infection, lower lobe predominance

*Hypercalcemia*

*Mitral stenosis* — Left atrial enlargement, may include valve calcification

*Alveolar microlithiasis* — Idiopathic with familial tendency; diffuse tiny (<1 mm) pulmonary calcifications

*Parasites* — *Dirofilaria immitis*

*Metastatic calcification* — Hyperparathyroidism

| | |
|---|---|
| *Amyloidosis* | Variable appearance including interstitial disease and solitary or multiple nodules, ± calcification or cavitation |
| *Calcified metastases* | Post–radiation therapy; mucinous adenocarcinoma from breast or colon; osteosarcoma; chondrosarcoma; cystosarcoma phyllodes; papillary adenocarcinoma from ovary or thyroid |

# INTERSTITIAL LUNG DISEASE
## 34. DIFFUSE INTERSTITIAL LUNG DISEASE

### Acute

**Pulmonary edema**	CHF, valvular heart disease, fluid overload, renal failure

**Pneumonia**	*Pneumocystis carinii; Mycoplasma;* viral—mononucleosis; *H. influenzae;* granulomatous disease—mycobacterial, fungus; viral—Rocky Mountain spotted fever

### Chronic

**Fibrosis**	Nodular thickening with architectural distortion, cystic airspaces, and traction bronchiectasis; idiopathic; drugs; connective tissue disease; asbestosis; chronic pneumonia; sarcoidosis

**Lymphangitic carcinomatosis**	Nodular interstitial process ± peribronchovascular and subpleural thickening and

| | |
|---|---|
| | effusion; breast and lung most common, also stomach, pancreas, and leukemia |
| Lymphocytic interstitial pneumonia | Idiopathic pseudolymphomatous condition most common in children with AIDS; septal thickening and ill-defined nodules |
| Sarcoidosis | Widely variable pulmonary patterns ± adenopathy including interstitial thickening and ill-defined nodules |
| Hypersensitivity pneumonitis | Immunologic response to inhaled organic antigens; small nodules, ground-glass appearance and septal lines that clear over weeks; chronic exposure leads to fibrosis |
| Eosinophilic granuloma | Upper lobe–predominant interstitial disease with a variable combination of small nodules and cysts; fibrosis and pneumothorax may develop |

## 90 LUNG

| | |
|---|---|
| *Leukemia and lymphoma* | Direct perihilar lymphatic spread can occur; usually associated with mediastinal adenopathy |
| *Pneumoconiosis silicosis* | |
| *Lymphangiectasia* | Rare, generalized lymphatic dilatation, small effusions |
| *Lymphangioleiomyomatosis and tuberous sclerosis* | Uniformly distributed thin-walled cysts in young women; pneumothorax and chylous effusion common complications; tuberous sclerosis can appear similar |
| *Idiopathic pulmonary hemosiderosis* | Recurrent pulmonary hemorrhage leads to septal thickening and eventual fibrosis |
| *Amyloidosis* | Interstitial disease and nodules ± calcification or cavitation |

## 35. NODULAR INTERSTITIAL DISEASE

**Pulmonary fibrosis**
Nodular thickening with architectural distortion, cystic airspaces, and traction bronchiectasis
Idiopathic (IPF)—DIP, UIP
End-stage lung disease (eosinophilic granuloma, sarcoidosis, silicosis)
Drugs—bleomycin, BCNU amiodarone, nitrofurantoin, methysergide, procainamide, busulfan, cyclophosphamide, methotrexate
Asbestosis—often seen associated pleural plaques
Connective tissue disease—scleroderma (thickened soft tissues, esophageal dysmotility), lupus (small pleural and pericardial effusions), rheumatoid lung, dermatomyositis
Chronic pneumonia—often associated bronchiectasis

| | |
|---|---|
| **Infection** | Mycobacterial, fungal—histoplasmosis, viral—mononucleosis, mycoplasma, PCP |
| **Lymphangitic carcinomatosis** | Nodular interstitial process ± peribronchovascular and subpleural thickening and effusion; breast and lung most common, also stomach, pancreas, and leukemia |
| ARDS | Noncardiogenic edema following pulmonary or systemic injury |
| Pulmonary metastases | Thyroid, melanoma |
| Bronchoalveolar cell carcinoma | Disseminated at time of detection |
| Sarcoidosis | Widely variable pulmonary patterns ± adenopathy including interstitial thickening and ill-defined nodules |
| Leukemia and lymphoma | Uncommon pattern of direct perihilar lymphatic spread; usually mediastinal adenopathy |

| | |
|---|---|
| Hypersensitivity pneumonitis | Immunologic response to inhaled organic antigens; acutely—small nodules, ground-glass appearance and septal lines that clear over weeks; chronic exposure leads to fibrosis |
| Silicosis and coal worker's pneumoconiosis | Small upper lobe–predominant, frequently calcified nodules and septal thickening, may coalesce to PMF with bronchiectasis and honeycombing, calcified nodes common |
| Eosinophilic granuloma | Upper lobe–predominant interstitial disease with a variable combination of small nodules and cysts; fibrosis and pneumothorax may develop |
| *Lymphangiectasia* | Rare, generalized lymphatic dilatation, small effusions |
| *Idiopathic pulmonary hemosiderosis* | Recurrent pulmonary hemorrhage leads to septal thickening and eventual fibrosis |

| | |
|---|---|
| *Alveolar microlithiasis* | Idiopathic with familial tendency; diffuse tiny (<1 mm) pulmonary calcifications |
| *Amyloidosis* | Variable appearance including interstitial disease and nodules ± calcification or cavitation |

## 36. DIFFUSE INTERSTITIAL DISEASE WITH PLEURAL EFFUSION

| | |
|---|---|
| **Pulmonary edema** | CHF, renal failure |
| Collagen vascular disease | Lupus, rheumatoid |
| Lymphangitic carcinomatosis | Reticulonodular interstitial process ± peribronchovascular and subpleural thickening and effusion; breast and lung most common; also stomach, pancreas, and leukemia |
| *Lymphoma or leukemia* | Usually associated mediastinal adenopathy |
| *Pneumonia* | Viral, mycoplasmal |
| *Lymphangioleiomyomatosis* | Uniformly distributed thin-walled cysts in young women; pneumothorax and chylous effusion common; tuberous sclerosis can appear similar |

## 37. DIFFUSE INTERSTITIAL DISEASE WITH ADENOPATHY

| | |
|---|---|
| **Stage II sarcoidosis** | Variable pulmonary patterns including interstitial thickening and ill-defined nodules; peribronchovascular nodules on HRCT |
| **Lymphoma or leukemia** | Direct perihilar interstitial spread from lymph nodes or lyphatic obstruction |
| Silicosis and coal worker's pneumoconiosis | Small upper lobe–predominant, frequently calcified nodules and septal thickening, may coalesce to PMF, calcified nodes common; stannosis, berylliosis, and siderosis are similar |
| Infection | Fungal, tuberculosis |
| Lymphangitic carcinomatosis | Nodular interstitial process ± peribronchovascular and subpleural thickening and effusion; breast and lung most common; also stomach, pancreas, and leukemia |

Idiopathic pulmonary fibrosis

Cystic fibrosis

# AIRSPACE DISEASE
## 38. FOCAL OR MULTIFOCAL CONSOLIDATION

**Infection**

**Bacterial** — *Pseudomonas; Staphylococcus aureus;* anaerobes—oral flora; *H. influenzae; Streptococcus*—usually lobar, effusion common; *Klebsiella*—usually lobar, may have bulging fissure; *Legionella; Nocardia; Actinomyces*

**Aspiration** — Recurrent pneumonia from anaerobes and gram-negative organisms in superior LL and posterior UL; alcoholism; debilitation; neurologic disorder—stroke; esophageal disease—achalasia, stricture, Zenker diverticulum, tumor; neuromuscular disease; TE fistula

| | |
|---|---|
| **Postobstructive** | Mucus plug, bronchogenic carcinoma, foreign body |
| Mycoplasma | |
| Mycobacterial | Tuberculosis |
| Fungal | Cryptococcosis, histoplasmosis |
| Lung abscess | Ill-defined cavity |
| *Eosinophilic pneumonia* | Loeffler syndrome, chronic eosinophilic pneumonia |

**Other causes**

| | |
|---|---|
| Atelectasis or collapse | Obstructive—endobronchial lesion; cicatrizing—fibrosis; compressive—bullae; passive—effusion |
| Hemorrhage | Focal or diffuse; bronchitis; bronchiectasis; pulmonary embolism; carcinoma; contusion; vasculitis—Wegener, Goodpasture, lupus; aspergilloma; anticoagulation; bleeding diathesis; AVM; DIC; metastases |
| Pulmonary infarct | Pleural-based, wedge-shaped; may include mosaic |

| | |
|---|---|
| | perfusion, emboli, volume loss, or effusion |
| Bronchoalveolar cell carcinoma | Mimics pneumonia; can present as focal or multifocal consolidation, nodules, or a mass |
| Sarcoidosis | Widely variable pulmonary patterns ± adenopathy including ill-defined nodules and occasional alveolar pattern |
| Radiation pneumonitis | Follows radiation port margins |
| *Lipoid pneumonia* | Chronic oil aspiration, areas of fat density |
| *Lymphoma* | Most commonly recurrent non-Hodgkin, usually mediastinal adenopathy; ill-defined nodules ± air bronchograms |
| *Pulmonary sequestration* | Congenital malformation with systemic arterial supply; LLL most common |

BOOP

Wegener granulomatosis

# 39. NODULAR AIRSPACE DISEASE

| | |
|---|---|
| **Sarcoidosis** | Variable pulmonary patterns ± adenopathy including ill-defined nodules |
| **Granulomatous disease** | Usually focal; histoplasmosis—small pulmonary nodules with calcification and frequently calcified mediastinal lymph nodes; tuberculosis |
| Aspiration pneumonia | Lower lobe and posterior upper lobes; alcoholism; debilitation; neurologic disorder—stroke; esophageal disease—achalasia, stricture, Zenker diverticula, tumor; neuromuscular disease; TE fistula |
| Lung cancer | Bronchoalveolar cell carcinoma |
| Lymphoma | Most commonly recurrent non-Hodgkin, ill-defined nodules ± air bronchograms, usually mediastinal adenopathy; direct perihilar lymphatic spread can occur |

| | |
|---|---|
| *Extrinsic allergic alveolitis* | Immunologic response to inhaled organic antigens; chronic exposure leads to fibrosis |

## 40. CHRONIC CONSOLIDATION

| | |
|---|---|
| **Bronchoalveolar cell carcinoma** | Can present as focal or multifocal consolidation, nodules, or a mass |
| **Postobstructive pneumonia** | "Drowned lung," bronchogenic carcinoma, foreign body, endobronchial metastasis |
| Fungal infection | Histoplasmosis, aspergillosis |
| Mycobacterial | Particularly tuberculosis, MAI, *M. kansasii* |
| *Eosinophilic pneumonia* | Loeffler syndrome, chronic eosinophilic pneumonia |
| *Lymphoma* | Most commonly recurrent non-Hodgkin, usually mediastinal adenopathy; variable pulmonary patterns including ill-defined nodules ± air bronchograms |
| *Lipoid pneumonia* | Chronic oil aspiration, areas of fat density |
| *Pulmonary sequestration* | Congenital malformation with systemic arterial supply, LLL most common; |

| | |
|---|---|
| | intralobar—pulmonary venous drainage, often discovered incidentally in adulthood; extralobar—less common, presents in infancy with infection, systemic venous drainage |
| *Cystic adenomatoid malformation* | |

## Recurrent pneumonia

| | |
|---|---|
| **Bronchial narrowing or obstruction** | Bronchogenic carcinoma; mucus plug; carcinoid; foreign body; broncholith; endobronchial metastasis; extrinsic mass |
| **Bronchiectasis** | Enlarged, thickened bronchi from chronic inflammation; cylindrical, varicose, and cystic patterns |
| **Repeated aspiration** | Recurrent pneumonia from anaerobes and gram-negative organisms, lower lobe and posterior upper lobes; alcoholism; debilitation; neurologic disorder—stroke; |

| | |
|---|---|
| | esophageal disease—achalasia, stricture, tumor, Zenker diverticula; neuromuscular disease; TE fistula |
| Immuno-compromised | HIV, AIDS, chemotherapy, malignancy |
| Cystic fibrosis | Autosomal recessive; hyperinflation, upper lobe–predominant bronchiectasis and mucus plugging, variable adenopathy; sinus disease and pancreatic insufficiency |
| Inadequate treatment | Ineffective or inadequate antibiotic course |

## 41. DIFFUSE PULMONARY CONSOLIDATION

**Pulmonary edema**
CHF, valvular heart disease, fluid overload, renal failure

**Broncho-pneumonia**
*Pseudomonas; Staphylococcus;* anaerobes; *Streptococcus; Klebsiella; Mycoplasma; Legionella; Nocardia; Actinomyces;* tuberculosis; viral; fungal—histoplasmosis, *Aspergillus;* lipoid—chronic oil aspiration

**Noncardiogenic edema—ARDS**
Trauma—burns, shock; sepsis; aspiration—Mendelson syndrome; pancreatitis; viral pneumonia; near-drowning; contusion; toxic inhalation—smoke, dust, gas (nitrogen dioxide, chlorine, hydrocarbon, phosgene); oxygen toxicity; DIC; multiple transfusions; drug reaction or overdose—morphine, heroin, cocaine, aspirin, TCA; sickle cell;

| | |
|---|---|
| | uremia; neurogenic—trauma, tumor, stroke; high altitude |
| **Pulmonary hemorrhage** | Focal or diffuse; bronchitis; bronchiectasis; pulmonary embolism; carcinoma; contusion; vasculitis—Wegener, Goodpasture, lupus; aspergilloma; anticoagulation; bleeding diathesis; AVM; DIC; metastases |
| Bronchoalveolar cell carcinoma | Can present as multifocal consolidation |
| BOOP | Bronchiolitis obliterans with organizing pneumonia—typically peripheral |
| Eosinophilic pneumonia | Chronic eosinophilic pneumonia; Loeffler syndrome—acute form |
| Lymphoma | Variable pattern, non-Hodgkin most commonly; usually associated mediastinal adenopathy |
| Hypersensitivity pneumonitis | Immunologic response to inhaled organic antigens, small nodules, ground-glass |

| | |
|---|---|
| | appearance; patchy consolidation and septal lines that clear over weeks |
| Alveolar proteinosis | Idiopathic overproduction or decreased absorption of surfactant by pneumocytes; diffuse, symmetric airspace disease ± septal thickening; treatment with BAL; predisposed to infection, particularly *Nocardia* |
| Radiation pneumonitis | Generally confined to radiation portal |
| *Sarcoidosis* | Uncommon pattern, ± adenopathy |
| *Amyloidosis* | Interstitial disease and solitary or multiple nodules, sometimes with calcification or cavitation |
| *Pulmonary embolism* | Fat, amniotic fluid, septic, bland thrombus |

## 42. PULMONARY HEMORRHAGE

**Bronchitis** — Thick-walled, nondilated bronchi, often radiographically occult

**Bronchiectasis** — Enlarged, thickened bronchi from chronic inflammation; cylindrical, varicose, and cystic patterns; focal type is often idiopathic; diffuse type from cystic fibrosis or immotile cilia syndrome; immune deficiency

**Pulmonary contusion** — Caused by blunt or penetrating chest trauma; resolves over days; often associated rib fracture

Impaired coagulation — Anticoagulation, thrombocytopenia, drugs, DIC, hemophilia, leukemia

Bronchogenic carcinoma — Irregular or spiculated mass; adenocarcinoma, squamous cell, large cell undifferentiated, bronchoalveolar; often metastasized to mediastinal nodes at presentation

| | |
|---|---|
| Iatrogenic | Bronchoscopy, biopsy |
| Sarcoidosis | Advanced disease with pulmonary fibrosis |
| Pulmonary embolism | May include areas of mosaic perfusion, intravascular emboli, volume loss or effusion |
| Vasculitis | Wegener granulomatosis, Goodpasture syndrome, lupus, others |
| Aspergilloma | Fungus ball eroding wall in preexisting cavity |
| AVM | Smooth, often multiple, feeding artery and draining vein |
| *Mitral stenosis* | Left atrial enlargement, usually valve calcification |
| *Idiopathic pulmonary hemosiderosis* | Recurrent pulmonary hemorrhage leads to septal thickening and eventual fibrosis |

# HRCT PATTERNS
## 43. GROUND-GLASS OPACITIES*

| | |
|---|---|
| **Pulmonary edema** | Smooth septal thickening |
| **Fibrosing alveolitis** | DIP, UIP—inflammatory phase of IPF |
| Hemorrhage | Focal or diffuse; bronchitis; bronchiectasis; pulmonary embolism; carcinoma; contusion; vasculitis—Wegener, Goodpasture, lupus; aspergilloma; anticoagulation; bleeding diathesis; AVM; DIC; metastases |
| Connective tissue disease | Particularly lupus |
| *Sarcoidosis* | Widely variable pulmonary involvement ± adenopathy including interstitial, nodular, and occasional alveolar pattern; peribronchovascular nodules on HRCT |

\* Partial airspace filling or alveolar septal inflammation that does not obscure vessels. Typically represents an active, acute, and reversible disease process.

| | |
|---|---|
| *Alveolar proteinosis* | Idiopathic overproduction of surfactant by pneumocytes; diffuse, symmetric airspace disease ± septal thickening; treatment with BAL; predisposed to infection, particularly *Nocardia* |
| *Eosinophilic granuloma* | Upper lobe–predominant interstitial disease with a variable combination of small nodules and cysts; fibrosis and pneumothorax may develop |

## Infection or Inflammation

| | |
|---|---|
| **Bacterial** | Alveolitis |
| **Viral** | Acute interstitial pneumonitis; CMV (often associated consolidation) |
| ***Pneumocystis carinii* pneumonia** | Common AIDS infection; perihilar interstitial or ground-glass pattern early; airspace, nodules, cysts, and pneumothorax when advanced; effusion and adenopathy rare; BAL usually diagnostic |

| | |
|---|---|
| Hypersensitivity pneumonitis | Immunologic response to inhaled organic antigens such as moldy hay or bird droppings; bilateral small nodules, ground-glass opacities, and patchy consolidation and septal lines that clear over weeks |
| BOOP | Typically peripheral, consolidation |
| Mycobacterial | Tuberculosis, MAI; centrilobular—"tree-in-bud" nodules |
| Bronchiolitis obliterans | Small airway inflammation; small centrilobular nodules, and "tree-in-bud" opacities on HRCT; air trapping on expiration |
| Eosinophilic pneumonia | Usually associated consolidation |
| *Lymphocytic interstitial pneumonia* | Idiopathic pseudolymphomatous condition in children with AIDS; septal thickening and ill-defined nodules |

## 44. SEPTAL THICKENING*

**Pulmonary edema**
Smooth, often associated areas of ground-glass opacity

**Pulmonary fibrosis**
Nodular thickening with architectural distortion and traction bronchiectasis, idiopathic, drug-related, connective tissue disease, sarcoidosis, asbestosis, chronic pneumonia

**Lymphangitic carcinomatosis**
Interstitial nodules ± peribronchovascular and subpleural thickening and effusion; breast and lung most common, also stomach, pancreas, and leukemia

**Hypersensitivity pneumonitis**
Immunologic response to inhaled organic antigens; bilateral small nodules, ground-glass opacities, patchy consolidation and septal lines acutely; chronic exposure leads to fibrosis

* Fluid or cellular infiltrates in interlobular septa. Linear opacities (1 to 2 cm) seen best in lung periphery. Visualization of a few peripheral interlobular septa is normal.

| | |
|---|---|
| Lymphoma | Uncommon pattern of direct perihilar lymphatic spread |
| Pneumonia | Viral—symmetric perihilar interstitial infiltrate, no effusion; mycoplasma |
| Sarcoidosis | Widely variable pulmonary patterns including interstitial thickening and 2- to 10-mm nodules ± adenopathy |
| Alveolar proteinosis | Idiopathic overproduction of surfactant by pneumocytes; diffuse, airspace disease ± septal thickening; treatment with BAL; predisposed to infection, particularly *Nocardia* |
| *Lymphangiectasia* | Rare, generalized lymphatic dilatation, small effusions |
| *Silicosis or coal worker's pneumoconiosis* | Small upper lobe–predominant, frequently calcified nodules and septal thickening, may coalesce to PMF with honeycombing, calcified nodes common |

## 45. PERIBRONCHOVASCULAR INTERSTITIAL THICKENING

**Pulmonary edema** — Smooth interstitial thickening with cardiomegaly and pleural effusions

**Sarcoidosis** — Widely variable pulmonary patterns including interstitial thickening and peribronchovascular nodules ± adenopathy

Lymphangitic carcinomatosis — Nodular, local spread of lung or hematogenous spread of breast cancer are most common

Kaposi sarcoma — Lower lobe bronchovascular thickening, skin or mucous membrane lesions invariably present

Lymphoma — Smooth or nodular; usually associated mediastinal adenopathy

Fibrosing alveolitis — UIP, DIP, IPF-associated traction bronchiectasis

| | |
|---|---|
| *Silicosis and coal worker's pneumoconiosis* | Small upper lobe–predominant, frequently calcified 2- to 5-mm nodules and septal thickening, may coalesce to PMF, calcified nodes common; stannosis, berylliosis, and siderosis are similar |
| *Hypersensitivity pneumonitis* | Immunologic response to inhaled organic antigens; acutely—small nodules, ground-glass opacities, patchy consolidation and septal lines that clear over weeks; chronic exposure leads to fibrosis |

## 46. SMALL NODULAR OPACITIES*

**Infection**

| | |
|---|---|
| **Broncho-pneumonia** | Ill-defined focal consolidation; *Pseudomonas; Staphylococcus;* anaerobes; *Streptococcus; Klebsiella; Mycoplasma; Legionella; Nocardia; Actinomyces;* tuberculosis; virus; fungal—histoplasmosis, aspergillosis; lipoid—chronic oil aspiration |
| **Old granulomatous disease** | Often calcified; histoplasmosis, tuberculosis |
| **Mycobacterial infection** | Transbronchial or hematogenous spread, particularly miliary tuberculosis |
| Bronchiolitis obliterans | Small airway inflammation; ground-glass attenuation, small centrilobular nodules, and "tree-in-bud" opacities on HRCT; expiratory images may show characteristic air trapping |

* Usually interstitial.

| | |
|---|---|
| Hypersensitivity pneumonitis | Immunologic response to inhaled organic antigens such as moldy hay or bird droppings; patterns include bilateral small nodules, ground-glass opacities, patchy consolidation, and septal lines |
| Lymphocytic interstitial pneumonia | Idiopathic pseudolymphomatous condition in children with AIDS; septal thickening and ill-defined centrilobular, peribronchovascular, and septal nodules |

### Tumors

| | |
|---|---|
| **Pulmonary metastases** | Smooth, round, various size lower lobe– and peripheral-predominant nodules; ill defined if hemorrhagic |
| **Lymphangitic carcinomatosis** | Nodular interstitial process ± peribronchovascular and subpleural thickening and effusion; breast and lung common; also stomach, pancreas, and leukemia |

| | |
|---|---|
| Bronchoalveolar cell carcinoma | Can present as focal or multifocal consolidation, nodules, or a mass |
| *Lymphoma* | Most commonly recurrent non-Hodgkin, almost always mediastinal adenopathy; nodules ± air bronchograms |

## Other causes

| | |
|---|---|
| **Sarcoidosis** | Widely variable pulmonary patterns ± adenopathy including interstitial thickening, ill-defined nodules; characteristic peribronchovascular nodules on HRCT |
| Eosinophilic granuloma | Upper lobe–predominant interstitial disease with a variable combination of small nodules and cysts; fibrosis and pneumothorax may develop |
| Silicosis and coal worker's pneumoconiosis | Small upper lobe– and posterior-predominant, frequently calcified nodules and septal thickening, may |

|  |  |
|---|---|
|  | coalesce to PMF, calcified nodes common |
| *Amyloidosis* | Variable, including interstitial disease and solitary or multiple nodules, ± calcification or cavitation |

## 47. SMALL NODULE DISTRIBUTION ON HRCT

| | |
|---|---|
| **<u>Perilymphatic</u>** | Peribronchovascular, septal, and subpleural |
| **Sarcoidosis** | Widely variable pulmonary patterns ± adenopathy including 2- to 10-mm peribronchovascular and subpleural nodules |
| **Lymphangitic carcinomatosis** | Interstitial nodular thickening (beaded septum) ± effusion; breast and lung common; also stomach, pancreas, and leukemia |
| Silicosis and coal worker's pneumoconiosis | Upper lobe– and posterior-predominant, frequently calcified nodules (2 to 5 mm) and septal thickening, may coalesce to PMF, calcified nodes common |
| *Lymphoma* | Usually associated mediastinal adenopathy |
| *Amyloidosis* | Solitary or multiple ± calcification or cavitation |

| | |
|---|---|
| *Lymphocytic interstitial pneumonia* | Idiopathic pseudolymphomatous condition in children with AIDS; septal thickening and ill-defined nodules |
| **Randomly distributed** | Evenly distributed throughout lung |
| Miliary tuberculosis | Typically very ill or immunocompromised patient |
| Fungal infection | Histoplasmosis, coccidiomycosis |
| Pulmonary metastases | Smooth, round, variable size, peripheral- and lower lobe–predominant; hemorrhagic nodules ill defined |

**Centrilobular**

| | |
|---|---|
| **Airway inflammation** | Bronchopneumonia; hypersensitivity pneumonitis—ill-defined nodules and ground-glass attenuation; bronchiectasis; cystic fibrosis—hyperinflation, bronchiectasis, |

|  |  |
|---|---|
|  | and mucus plugging; allergic bronchopulmonary aspergillosis, asthma |
| **Bronchiolitis** | Ground-glass and "tree-in-bud" opacities; expiratory images may show air trapping in involved regions |
| **Mycobacterial infection** | Endobronchial spread of tuberculosis or MAI; "tree-in-bud" pattern |
| Bronchoalveolar cell carcinoma | Can present as focal or multifocal consolidation, nodules, or a mass |
| Eosinophilic granuloma | Upper lobe–predominant interstitial disease with a variable combination of small nodules and cysts; fibrosis and pneumothorax may develop |

# PLEURA

## 48. PNEUMOTHORAX

### Trauma

**Iatrogenic**  Thoracentesis, surgery, percutaneous or transbronchial biopsy, CVL or pacemaker placement

**Barotrauma (volotrauma)**  Often preceded by pneumomediastinum; positive-pressure ventilation

**Accidents**  Rib fracture; closed chest trauma; penetrating injury; tracheobronchial injury

Esophageal rupture  Endoscopy, cancer, spontaneous—Boerhaave syndrome

Dissection  From pneumoperitoneum or pneumomediastinum

### Focal lung disease

**Ruptured cystic airspace**  Bulla or bleb—tall, thin men; pneumatocele, emphysema, asthma, cystic fibrosis, PCP, eosinophilic granuloma, lymphangioleiomyomatosis

| | |
|---|---|
| Bronchogenic carcinoma | Irregular or spiculated mass, often metastasized to mediastinal nodes at presentation |
| Necrotizing pneumonia or ruptured abscess | *Staphylococcus*, tuberculosis |

## Diffuse lung disease

| | |
|---|---|
| **Cystic fibrosis** | Autosomal recessive; hyperinflation, upper lobe–predominant bronchiectasis, variable adenopathy; sinus disease and pancreatic insufficiency |
| ***Pneumocystis carinii* pneumonia** | Pneumothorax is often difficult to treat; perihilar interstitial or ground-glass pattern; airspace, nodular, cysts, and pneumothorax in advanced disease |
| **Asthmatic attack** | Pneumomediastinum is more common |
| Pulmonary fibrosis | Septal thickening with architectural distortion, traction bronchiectasis, |

and ground-glass opacities; idiopathic, drug-related, connective tissue disease, asbestosis, chronic pneumonia

*Pulmonary metastases* — Particularly osteosarcoma

*Lymphangio-leiomyomatosis* — Uniformly distributed thin-walled cysts in young women; pneumothorax and chylous effusion common complications; tuberous sclerosis can appear similar

Eosinophilic granuloma — Upper lobe–predominant interstitial disease with a variable combination of small nodules and cysts; fibrosis and pneumothorax may develop

## **Pleural**

Bronchopleural fistula — Prolonged air leak following pulmonary surgery or pneumonia

*Catamenial* — Endometriosis

# 49. TYPES OF PLEURAL FLUID

| | |
|---|---|
| **Transudate** | (Protein < 3 g/dl) |
| **Congestive heart failure, renal failure, fluid overload** | Cardiomegaly, pulmonary vascular enlargement, and pulmonary edema dependent on severity; effusions (right > left) |
| Nephrotic syndrome | Diffuse body-wall edema |
| Cirrhosis | Effusion secondary to hypoproteinemia with systemic edema or transgression of ascites across diaphragm |
| Ascites | Peritoneal dialysis, other causes |
| *SVC obstruction* | Bronchogenic carcinoma, fibrosing mediastinitis, central venous catheter induced |
| *Myxedema* | Hyperthyroidism |

| | |
|---|---|
| *Constrictive pericarditis* | Thickened fibrous pericardium, right heart failure |
| **Exudate** | (Protein > 3 g/dl) |
| **Parapneumonic effusion** | Bacteria, tuberculosis |
| **Malignant effusion** | Pleural metastases, bronchogenic carcinoma, lymphoma, leukemia, mesothelioma |
| Collagen vascular | Particularly lupus |
| Dressler syndrome | Recent cardiac surgery or MI, elevated sedimentation rate, chest pain |
| *Meig syndrome* | Pleural effusion and ascites associated with benign ovarian fibroma |
| Miscellaneous | Pulmonary thromboembolism, subphrenic abscess, drug induced, pericardial disease, postpartum |

## TYPES OF PLEURAL FLUID 133

| | |
|---|---|
| **<u>Hemothorax</u>** | High attenuation on CT |
| **Chest trauma** | Torn intercostal vessel, rib fracture or contusion may be seen |
| **Iatrogenic** | Central venous catheter placement, thoracentesis, chest tube placement, percutaneous lung biopsy |
| **Malignancy** | Bronchogenic carcinoma, pleural metastases, mesothelioma |
| Torn pleural adhesion | Most common spontaneous cause |
| Coagulopathy | Anticoagulation, hemophilia |
| *Uncommon* | Catamenial—endometriosis; dissecting aortic aneurysm; hematopiesis—paraspinal soft tissue, expanded ribs |
| **<u>Chylothorax</u>** | (High lipid content, may be less dense than water on CT) |
| **Traumatic injury to thoracic duct** | Cardiothoracic surgery; penetrating and closed injuries; may take months to develop; low injury—right |

| | |
|---|---|
| | effusion; high injury—left effusion |
| Lymphoma | Almost always associated mediastinal adenopathy |
| *Lymphangioleiomyomatosis* | Uniformly distributed thin-walled cysts in young women; pneumothorax and chylous effusion common; tuberous sclerosis can appear similar |
| *Lymphangioma* | Cystic hygroma; benign congenital lymphatic malformation; neck >> mediastinum |
| *Uncommon* | Metastatic disease; mediastinal fibrosis; central venous obstruction; tumor invasion; filariasis; left subclavian vein thrombosis; congenital lymphangiectasia |

# 50. UNILATERAL PLEURAL EFFUSION

## Cardiovascular

**Congestive heart failure** — Cardiomegaly, pulmonary vascular enlargement, edema; septal and fissural thickening, airspace fluid dependent on severity; pleural effusions (right > left)

**Pulmonary embolism** — Mosaic perfusion may be seen, as well as intravascular emboli, volume loss, or effusion; infarcts appear as pleural-based, wedge-shaped opacities

**Recent chest surgery** — Left effusion invariably follows cardiac surgery

Dressler syndrome — Recent cardiac surgery or MI, elevated sedimentation rate, chest pain; effusion (left > right)

## Inflammatory

**Parapneumonic effusion** — Associated lung disease; bacteria—*Staphylococcus,*

|  |  |
|---|---|
|  | *Streptococcus, Klebsiella; Mycoplasma,* fungal, viral, parasitic, protozoan, mycobacterial—may lack associated lung disease with tuberculosis |
| Pericarditis | Viral, idiopathic, tuberculosis, metastatic |
| Abdominal | Pyelonephritis; pancreatitis (left > right); subphrenic abscess—postoperative |
| Radiation therapy | Serous fluid |

**Malignant**

|  |  |
|---|---|
| **Pleural metastases** | Breast, lung, lymphoma, ovarian, stomach, pancreas, renal |
| Bronchogenic carcinoma | Direct extension to pleura |
| Mesothelioma | Plaques ± calcification from asbestos exposure in 50% |
| Lymphoma or leukemia | Usually associated mediastinal adenopathy |

## **Traumatic**

| | |
|---|---|
| Vascular injury | Catheter placement, hemothorax |
| Pulmonary contusion or laceration | Blunt or penetrating chest trauma; resolves over days; often associated rib fracture |
| Esophageal rupture or fistula | Cancer, dilatation, endoscopy, oral or gastric contents, left ≥ right |
| Thoracic duct rupture | Chylothorax, low—right effusion; high—left effusion |

## 51. BILATERAL PLEURAL EFFUSIONS

**Congestive heart failure, fluid overload** — Cardiomegaly, pulmonary vascular enlargement and pulmonary edema dependent on severity; effusions (right > left)

**Pleural metastases** — Breast, lung, lymphoma, ovarian, stomach, pancreas, renal

**Recent chest surgery** — Reactive effusions

Collagen vascular disease — Usually small, often associated lung disease; lupus, rheumatoid

Leukemia or lymphoma — Usually associated mediastinal adenopathy

Drugs — Nitrofurantoin, methysergide, methotrexate

Asbestos exposure — Usually small, pleural plaques often seen

*Uncommon* — Pericarditis, myxedema, Dressler syndrome (left > right)

## Abdominal disease

| | |
|---|---|
| **Renal failure** | Uremia, often with edema |
| Ascites | Peritoneal dialysis (see Differential 76) |
| Hypoproteinemia | Systemic edema, ascites; cirrhosis, nephrotic syndrome, malnutrition |
| Pancreatitis | Left >> right |
| *Meig syndrome* | Pleural effusion and ascites associated with benign ovarian fibroma |

## 52. PLEURAL EFFUSION WITH CARDIOMEGALY

**Congestive heart failure** — Cardiomegaly and pulmonary vascular enlargement with edema; septal and fissural thickening progressing to airspace disease; effusions (right > left)

Pulmonary embolism — Areas of mosaic perfusion may be seen, as well as intravascular emboli, volume loss, or effusion; infarcts appear as pleural-based wedge-shaped opacities

### Associated pericardial effusion

Pericarditis — Pericardial thickening, effusion

Lupus — Serositis, occasional pneumonitis

Dressler syndrome — Recent cardiac surgery or MI, elevated sedimentation rate, chest pain (left > right)

Lymphoma and leukemia — Usually associated mediastinal adenopathy

*Metastases* — Pleural and pericardial metastases from breast or lung

## 53. PLEURAL THICKENING

| | |
|---|---|
| **Extrapleural fat deposition** | Symmetric fat density; obesity, steroid use |
| **Asbestos exposure** | Often calcified, usually bilateral |
| Organized effusion | Prior surgery, hemorrhage, empyema |
| Prior empyema | Particularly tuberculosis |
| Pulmonary fibrosis | When advanced |
| Metastatic disease | Nodular; adenocarcinoma—breast, lung, stomach, pancreas, ovary, renal |
| Mesothelioma | May be focal or diffuse; typically lobulated |
| Fibrosing mediastinitis | Calcified lymph nodes and mediastinal fibrosis |

## 54. PLEURAL CALCIFICATIONS

| | |
|---|---|
| **Asbestos exposure** | Bilateral, symmetric; parietal pleura |
| **Prior empyema or hemothorax** | Unilateral, thick calcifications from tuberculosis, visceral pleura |
| Pleurodesis | Pleurodesis—talc may simulate calcification |
| *Uncommon* | Chronic hemodialysis, chronic pancreatitis; talcosis |

## 55. PLEURAL MASS

| | |
|---|---|
| **Loculated effusion** | Fluid density, smooth margins |
| **Pleural thickening or plaque** | Particularly from asbestos exposure; also prior infection, hemorrhage, or surgery |
| Empyema | "Split-pleura sign," follows pleural contour; displaces lung; *S. aureus; Pneumococcus; E. coli; Klebsiella; Pseudomonas;* anaerobes |
| *Thoracic splenosis* | Prior splenic and diaphragmatic trauma |

### Neoplasms

| | |
|---|---|
| **Peripheral lung cancer** | Superior sulcus tumor may simulate a pleural mass |
| **Lymphoma** | Paraspinal pleural involvement common, usually associated mediastinal adenopathy |
| **Extraosseous extension of rib lesion** | Metastasis, multiple myeloma |

| | |
|---|---|
| Extrapleural tumor | Neural—schwannoma, neurofibroma; lipoma, sarcoma, desmoid |
| Pleural metastases | Enhancing nodules, often associated effusion; adenocarcinoma—breast, lung, pancreas, ovary |
| Mesothelioma | Malignant tumor of pleura, strong association with asbestos exposure; plaques ± calcification seen in 50% |
| Invasive thymoma | Malignant anterior mediastinal mass; invasion of adjacent structures with pleural metastases can occur |
| *Fibrous tumor* | Benign, smooth, often pedunculated tumor attached to visceral pleura, may appear in fissure; may cause hypertrophic pulmonary osteoarthropathy or hypoglycemia |

## 56. MULTIPLE PLEURAL MASSES

| | |
|---|---|
| **Loculated effusions** | Fluid density, smooth, sharply marginated |
| **Pleural plaques** | Asbestos—usually bilateral, often calcified |
| **Pleural metastases** | Enhancing nodules, often associated effusion; adenocarcinoma—breast, lung |
| Mesothelioma | Malignant tumor of pleura, strong association with asbestos exposure; plaques ± calcification seen in 50% |
| Invasive thymoma | Malignant anterior mediastinal mass; invasion of adjacent structures with pleural metastases can occur |
| *Fibrous tumor* | Benign, smooth, often pedunculated tumor attached to visceral pleura, may appear in fissure; usually solitary |
| *Endometriosis* | May lead to catamenial pneumothorax |

| | |
|---|---|
| *Lymphoma* | Usually associated mediastinal adenopathy |
| *Thoracic splenosis* | Traumatic splenic injury with implantation of fragments that grow on vascular pleural surface, confirmed by sulfur colloid or heat damaged red blood cell scintigraphy |

## 57. EXTRAPLEURAL LESION

| | |
|---|---|
| **Lipoma** | Characteristic fat density |
| **Hematoma** | Rib fracture, surgery, catheter placement |
| **Rib metastasis or multiple myeloma** | Bone destruction with extraosseous soft tissue extension |
| Chest wall infection | Particularly tuberculosis, actinomycosis; *Nocardia*, blastomycosis |
| *Primary bone tumor* | Ewing sarcoma, chondrosarcoma |
| *Soft tissue tumor* | Dermoid, hemangioma, Askin tumor, fibroma |

# MEDIASTINUM AND HILA

## 58. PNEUMOMEDIASTINUM

| | |
|---|---|
| **Recent surgery** | Tracheostomy, sternotomy, pericardial drainage, neck dissection, esophagectomy |
| **Penetrating injury** | Gunshot, stabbing |
| **Extension from neck or abdomen** | Pneumoretroperitoneum or subcutaneous emphysema |
| **Volotrauma/ barotrauma** | Ventilated patient; stiff lungs—fibrosis |
| Tracheo-bronchial injury | Intubation, bronchoscopy, chest trauma |
| Esophageal tear | Endoscopy, dilatation, cancer, Boerhaave syndrome with "V sign of Naclerio" |
| Miscellaneous | Asthmatic attack, cough, vomiting, idiopathic, bronchial dihiscence post lung transplant |
| *Tracheal or esophageal fistula* | Tumor, infection |

## 59. UNILATERAL HILAR ENLARGEMENT

| | |
|---|---|
| **Central bronchogenic carcinoma** | Squamous cell, small cell |
| Bronchogenic cyst | Sharply marginated, fluid-filled mass, usually near carina; infection can lead to bronchial communication and air-fluid level |

### Adenopathy

| | |
|---|---|
| **Metastases** | Bronchogenic carcinoma, head and neck cancer, renal cell, testicular cancer |
| **Granulomatous infection** | Primary tuberculosis, histoplasmosis, coccidiomycosis |
| Reactive | Bacterial pneumonia or abscess, viral—mononucleosis; AIDS |
| *Lymphoma* | Rare without associated mediastinal adenopathy |
| *Sarcoidosis* | Almost always bilateral hilar adenopathy, often associated |

| | |
|---|---|
| | paratracheal, prevascular, or subcarinal nodes when advanced |
| *Castleman disease* | Angiofollicular lymph node hyperplasia—idiopathic; may compress adjacent structures; striking contrast enhancement ± calcification |

## Pulmonary artery

| | |
|---|---|
| Pulmonary stenosis | Main and left pulmonary artery enlargement, normal right pulmonary artery |
| Prior surgical systemic to pulmonary shunt | Blalock-Taussig, Waterston-Cooley, Potts-Smith |
| *Pseudoaneurysm* | Overinflation of pulmonary artery catheter, tuberculosis (Rasmussin) |
| *Congenital* | Congenital absence of the pulmonary valve—often associated with tetralogy of Fallot |

## 60. BILATERAL HILAR ENLARGEMENT

### Vascular

**Pulmonary artery hypertension** — Fibrosis, interstitial disease, emphysema, pulmonary emboli, idiopathic, left-to-right shunt

Normal variant — Pulmonary artery dilatation may be normal in young adult

Venous engorgement — Mitral valve disease, congestive heart failure, TAPVR below the diaphragm, left atrial myxoma

*Left-to-right shunt* — Patent ductus arteriosus, ASD, VSD

*High-output heart disease* — Anemia, thyrotoxicosis, pregnancy, AVMs

### Adenopathy

**Sarcoidosis** — Bilateral hilar and often paratracheal, prevascular, or subcarinal adenopathy ± associated lung disease

| | |
|---|---|
| **Granulomatous infection** | Tuberculosis, histoplasmosis, coccidiomycosis |
| **Metastases** | Bronchogenic, head and neck, renal cell, testicular primaries |
| Lymphoma or leukemia | Often asymmetric |
| Reactive | Bacterial pneumonia or abscess; viral—mononucleosis; AIDS |
| *Cystic fibrosis* | Hyperinflation, upper lobe–predominant bronchiectasis, and variable adenopathy |
| *Silicosis* | Calcified nodes common, sometimes with eggshell pattern; small upper lobe–predominant, frequently calcified nodules, which may coalesce to PMF |
| *Castleman disease* | Angiofollicular lymph node hyperplasia—idiopathic; may compress adjacent structures; striking contrast enhancement ± calcification |
| Kaposi sarcoma | AIDS, associated nodular bronchovascular thickening |

# 61. CARDIOPHRENIC ANGLE MASS

## Mediastinal

| | |
|---|---|
| **Fat** | Large pericardial fat pad |
| **Pericardial cyst** | Sharply marginated, fluid density, no enhancement, high protein content may produce higher density, right > left |
| **Enlarged right atrium** | ASD, right ventricular failure, tricuspid stenosis or insufficiency, endocardial cushion defect, anomalous pulmonary venous return, Ebstein anomaly |
| Mediastinal tumor | Thymoma, lymphoma, germ cell tumor |
| Pericardial effusion | Separation of visceral and parietal pericardium with outward displacement of pericardial fat |
| Left ventricular aneurysm | Prior myocardial infarction; often apical, sometimes calcified |

| | |
|---|---|
| Epicardial lymphadenopathy | Lymphoma, malignant thymoma, metastases |

## Pulmonary

| | |
|---|---|
| Peripheral lung mass | Bronchogenic carcinoma, sequestration |
| Pneumonia or collapse | May have air bronchograms |

## Abdominal

| | |
|---|---|
| **Stomach** | Hiatal hernia or esophagectomy with gastric interposition |
| Morgagni hernia | Herniation of fat, abdominal organs, or gastrointestinal tract through anteromedial parasternal diaphragm defect |
| *Ruptured hemidiaphragm* | Blunt or penetrating trauma; diagnosis often delayed |

## Pleural

| | |
|---|---|
| Loculated effusion | Sharply marginated fluid density |
| Pleural mass | Fibrous tumor, mesothelioma, mestastases |

## 62. ANTERIOR MEDIASTINAL MASS*

| | |
|---|---|
| **Thyroid mass** | May compress trachea or esophagus, goiter, adenoma, carcinoma |
| **Lymphoma** | Hodgkin disease more often than non-Hodgkin |
| **Thymic mass** | Thymoma—30% have myasthenia gravis; invasive or encapsulated; thymolipoma—contains fat; thymic carcinoma; rebound hyperplasia; thymic cyst—fluid density unless hemorrhage or infected; rarely thymic carcinoid |
| **Germ cell neoplasm** | Mature teratoma—often contain fat or bone; cystic are usually benign, solid generally malignant; seminoma; choriocarcinoma |
| **Fat deposition** | Obesity, steroids, lipoma |

* Bounded anteriorly by sternum and posteriorly by brachiocephalic vessels, aorta, and anterior pericardium.

| | |
|---|---|
| Vascular | Ascending aortic aneurysm; enlarged superior vena cava—elevated central venous pressure or obstruction; tortuous brachiocephalic vessels, valvular aortic stenosis, sinus of Valsalva aneurysm, right coronary artery aneurysm |
| Morgagni hernia | Herniation of fat, abdominal organs, or gastrointestinal tract through anteromedial diaphragm defect |
| Fluid collection | Postoperative or perforated central venous catheter |
| Inflammation | Median sternotomy, mediastinitis, fibrosing mediastinitis |
| Sternal mass | Metastasis—breast, multiple myeloma; Ewing sarcoma, chondrosarcoma |
| Hematoma | Posttraumatic |
| Pericardial cyst | Sharply marginated, fluid density, no enhancement, high protein content may |

|  |  |
|---|---|
|  | produce higher density, most common in right cardiophrenic angle |
| *Parathyroid mass* | Adenoma, carcinoma; usually small |
| *Lymphangioma* | Cystic hygroma; benign congenital lymphatic malformation; neck >> mediastinum |
| *Hemangioma* | Uncommonly with phleboliths |
| *Sarcoma* | Angiosarcoma, liposarcoma |

# 63. MIDDLE MEDIASTINAL MASS*

## Vascular

| | |
|---|---|
| **Ascending aortic aneurysm** | Poststenotic dilatation in aortic stenosis, Marfan syndrome, mycotic, atherosclerotic |
| Tortuous vessels | Brachiocephalic artery elongates and becomes ectatic with age; atherosclerotic calcification common |
| Pulmonary artery enlargement | Pulmonary artery hypertension; left-to-right shunt—ASD, VSD |
| Aortic arch | Right-sided or double |
| Left superior vena cava | Right-sided SVC may be normal or absent |

* Contains heart, ascending and transverse aorta, superior and inferior vena cava, brachiocephalic vessels, trachea and main bronchi, and central pulmonary arteries and veins.

| | |
|---|---|
| Enlarged azygos vein | CHF, SVC obstruction, elevated central venous pressure, azygos continuation of IVC (often associated with polysplenia), portal hypertension, Budd-Chiari |
| Aberrant vessel | Aberrant right subclavian artery passes behind esophagus; aberrant left pulmonary artery, partial anomalous pulmonary venous rectum, aberrant left brachiocephalic vein, left superior intercostal vein (aortic nipple) |

## Lymphadenopathy

| | |
|---|---|
| **Lymphoma** or leukemia | Particularly Hodgkin disease and CLL |
| **Bronchogenic carcinoma** | Particularly small cell |
| Extrathoracic malignancy | Renal cell, testicular, ovarian, head and neck, thyroid, breast, melanoma |
| Reactive | Lung abscess, tuberculosis, histoplasmosis, cystic fibrosis, mononucleosis, IPF |

| | |
|---|---|
| Silicosis | Calcified mediastinal nodes common, sometimes with an "eggshell" pattern; small upper lobe–predominant, frequently calcified nodules, may coalesce to PMF |
| *Sarcoidosis* | Almost always bilateral hilar adenopathy, often associated paratracheal, prevascular, or subcarinal nodes when advanced |
| *Castleman disease* | Angiofollicular lymph node hyperplasia—idiopathic; may compress adjacent structures; striking contrast enhancement and often calcification |

## Primary tumors

| | |
|---|---|
| Central bronchogenic cancer | Particularly small cell or squamous |
| Tracheal tumor | Squamous cell, adenoid cystic carcinoma, metastasis, may have large extraluminal component |

| | |
|---|---|
| Esophageal tumor | Leiomyoma, squamous cell, adenocarcinoma |
| Parathyroid tumor | Adenoma |
| *Cardiac tumor* | Myxoma, angiosarcoma |

**Other causes**

| | |
|---|---|
| **Duplication cyst** | Bronchogenic or esophageal; sharp margins, fluid density |
| Thyroid mass | Large goiter, often with calcification, can be retrotracheal |
| Morgagni hernia | Herniation of abdominal fat, upper abdominal organs, or GI tract through an anteromedial diaphragm defect |
| Pericardial cyst | Sharply marginated thin-walled fluid density mass adjacent to pericardium (R >> L) |
| Hematoma | Trauma, surgery |
| Fluid collection | Postoperative or perforated central venous catheter |

| | |
|---|---|
| Inflammation | Median sternotomy, mediastinitis, fibrosing mediastinitis |
| *Pancreatic pseudocyst* | Encapsulated fluid collection representing sequela of inflammation; some communicate with pancreatic duct; complications include hemorrhage and infection |

# 64. POSTERIOR MEDIASTINAL MASS*

## Spinal masses

| | |
|---|---|
| **Neurogenic tumor** | Schwannoma (neurilemoma), neurofibroma, neuroblastoma, neurofibrosarcoma, ganglioneuroma, ganglioneuroblastoma, malignant schwannoma |
| Paraganglioma | Chemodectoma, pheochromocytoma |
| Paraspinal abscess | Discitis, tuberculosis, *Staphylococcus* |
| *Hematoma* | Compression fracture |
| *Extramedullary hematopoiesis* | Anemia, often bilateral paraspinal masses |
| *Bone tumor involving spine or posterior ribs* | Primary or metastasis—renal, breast, multiple myeloma; Ewing sarcoma |

* Bounded by the posterior pericardium anteriorly, the paravertebral gutters posteriorly, and mediastinal pleura laterally.

| | |
|---|---|
| *Neuroenteric cyst* | Congenital, sharply defined, fluid-filled foregut cyst; vertebral anomalies |
| *Meningocele* | Spine or rib anomaly often seen |

## Gastrointestinal

| | |
|---|---|
| **Stomach** | Hiatal hernia or esophagectomy with gastric conduit |
| **Enlarged esophagus** | Achalasia, scleroderma, obstructing stricture or tumor |
| Esophageal duplication cyst or diverticulum | Fluid density, occasionally with air-fluid level |
| Esophageal tumor | Leiomyoma, squamous cell, adenocarcinoma |
| Bochdalek hernia | Usually posterolateral left-sided |
| *Pancreatic pseudocyst* | Encapsulated fluid collection from pancreatic inflammation; may communicate with pancreatic duct; complications include hemorrhage and infection |

| | |
|---|---|
| Fluid collection | Ascites, mediastinal extension through esophageal hiatus |

### Vascular

| | |
|---|---|
| **Aortic aneurysm** | Descending thoracic aorta |
| Enlarged azygos vein | CHF, SVC obstruction, elevated central venous pressure, azygos continuation of IVC (often associated with polysplenia), portal hypertension, Budd-Chiari |
| Paraesophageal varices | Portal venous hypertension from cirrhosis, venous thrombosis from pancreatitis |
| Hemangioma | Uncommonly with phleboliths |

### Paraspinal (pulmonary/pleural)

| | |
|---|---|
| Pleural thickening or loculated effusion | Sharply marginated fluid density |
| Lipoma | Fat density |
| Lymphoma | Usually associated anterior mediastinal adenopathy |

# 65. LOW-ATTENUATION MEDIASTINAL MASS

## Fat density

| | |
|---|---|
| **Fat deposition** | Obesity, steroids |
| Lipoma | Fat density |
| Thymolipoma | Benign tumor with fat and soft tissue density draped over anterior mediastinum |
| Mature teratoma | Often contains fat or bone; cystic is usually benign, solid is malignant |
| *Liposarcoma* | Variable fat and soft tissue components |

## Fluid density

| | |
|---|---|
| **Duplication cyst** | Bronchogenic or esophageal |
| **Fluid collection** | Seroma from trauma or surgery, perforated central venous catheter (rare) |
| **Pericardial cyst** | Most common in right cardiophrenic angle, sharp margins, thin wall |

## LOW-ATTENUATION MEDIASTINAL MASS

| | |
|---|---|
| Loculated pleural effusion | Sharply marginated, fluid density |
| Thymic cyst | Fluid density |
| Paraspinal abscess | Discitis, tuberculosis, *Staphylococcus* |
| Pancreatic pseudocyst | Encapsulated fluid collection representing sequelae of peripancreatic inflammation; some communicate with pancreatic duct; complications include hemorrhage and infection |
| *Meningocele* | Spine or rib anomaly often seen |
| *Neuroenteric cyst* | Congenital, sharply defined, fluid-filled foregut cyst associated with vertebral anomalies |
| *Lymphangioma* | Cystic hygroma; benign congenital lymphatic malformation, neck >> mediastinum |

| | |
|---|---|
| *Ascites* | Mediastinal extension through esophageal hiatus |

### Gastrointestinal

| | |
|---|---|
| **Stomach** | Hiatal hernia or esophagectomy with gastric interposition |
| Enlarged esophagus | Achalasia, scleroderma, obstruction from stricture or tumor, diverticulum |
| Morgagni hernia | Herniation of fat, abdominal organs, or gastrointestinal tract through an anteromedial diaphragm defect |
| Bochdalek hernia | Usually contains only fat, posterolateral, left > right |

# CARDIAC AND VASCULAR

# 66. CARDIOMEGALY

**Cardiomyopathy** Ischemic, viral, idiopathic, postpartum

## Left ventricle

| | |
|---|---|
| **Congestive heart failure** | Cardiomegaly and pulmonary vascular engorgement with edema; septal and fissural thickening progressing to airspace disease; fluid dependent on severity; pleural effusions (right > left) |
| **Ischemic heart disease** | Coronary artery calcifications may be seen; pulmonary edema with acute MI |
| **High-output heart disease** | Anemia, sickle cell disease, fluid overload, AV fistula, polycythemia vera, pregnancy, thyrotoxicosis |
| Valvular heart disease | Aortic or mitral insufficiency, AS—poststenotic dilatation of the aorta |
| Coarctation of the aorta | Typically postductal in adults, rib notching |

| | |
|---|---|
| Hypertension | May cause only left ventricular hypertrophy, not enlargement |
| Congenital heart disease | Truncus arteriosus, Ebstein anomaly, pulmonary atresia |

### Left atrium

| | |
|---|---|
| Mitral insufficiency | Left ventricular enlargement, due to rheumatic heart disease or papillary muscle dysfunction from CAD |
| Left-to-right shunts | Patent ductus arteriosus |
| *Left atrial myxoma* | Occasionally calcifies |

### Right ventricle

| | |
|---|---|
| **Cor pulmonale** | PA hypertension, enlarged PA, severe lung disease, pulmonary emboli, idiopathic |
| Atrial septal defect | Late finding; also see right atrial, PA, and venous enlargement |
| Valvular heart disease | Pulmonary or tricuspid insufficiency |

## Right atrium

| | |
|---|---|
| **Right ventricular failure** | Left ventricular failure is the most common cause of right ventricular failure |
| **Atrial septal defect** | Right ventricular and pulmonary artery enlargement |
| Tricuspid insufficiency | Associated IVC and hepatic vein enlargement; carcinoid syndrome, endocarditis in drug abusers |
| Tricuspid stenosis | Carcinoid syndrome, lupus, endomyocardial fibrosis, rheumatic heart disease, congenital |
| *Congenital heart disease* | Endocardial cushion defect—associated with Down syndrome; Ebstein anomaly—box-shaped heart, frequently associated with Wolff-Parkinson-White syndrome; PAPVR—anomalous draining vein |

## 67. CARDIAC MASS

| | |
|---|---|
| **Bland thrombus** | Left atrial in patients with atrial fibrillation or mitral valve disease; left ventricular within an aneurysm; dilated cardiomyopathy |
| **Primary benign tumor** | Myxoma—often pedunculated, attached to atrial septum, LA >> RA > RV location; atrial septal lipoma; rhabdomyoma—patient with tuberous sclerosis; fibroma; fibromyxoma; hamartoma |
| Tumor emboli | Renal cell, hepatoma, adrenal tumor |
| Direct invasion | Lymphoma, lung, esophagus, thymoma |
| *Metastases* | Carcinoid, breast, melanoma, lymphoma, lung, osteosarcoma, chondrosarcoma |
| *Primary malignant tumor* | Angiosarcoma, RA most common cardiac site |

## 68. PERICARDIAL EFFUSION

| | |
|---|---|
| **Idiopathic** | One-third of all cases |
| **Infectious pericarditis** | Tuberculosis, viral—coxsackievirus |
| Recent cardiac surgery | Coronary bypass or valve replacement most commonly |
| Collagen vascular disease | Lupus—often small chronic pleural effusions |
| Dressler syndrome | Effusion in 70%, fever, chest pain, pleural effusion or infiltrate, elevated sedimentation rate |
| Metabolic | Uremia, myxedema |
| Congestive heart failure | Cardiomegaly and pulmonary vascular engorgement with edema, pleural effusions |
| Tumor | Metastases—lymphoma, breast, melanoma, carcinoid; direct invasion—lung, cardiac, thymoma |
| *Radiation therapy* | Thickened pericardium |
| *Hemopericardium* | Aortic dissection, trauma, coagulopathy |

## 69. CARDIAC CALCIFICATIONS

| | |
|---|---|
| **Coronary arteries** | Correlates with severity of atherosclerosis and risk of MI but not location-specific |
| **Mitral annulus** | Usually clinically insignificant |
| **Aortic valve** | Bicuspid, rheumatic, endocarditis, atherosclerosis, predisposes to stenosis |
| **Pericardium** | Prior viral or tuberculous pericarditis often spares apex; rheumatic, syphilis, asbestos |
| Mitral valve | Rheumatic heart disease |
| Left atrium | Mitral valve disease |
| Myocardial | Aneurysm, old MI, commonly involves cardiac apex; syphilis, trauma |
| Ascending aorta | Hyperlipoproteinemia—homozygous type II; diabetes; syphilis—dense calcification, dilated; atherosclerotic |
| Left ventricular thrombus | Particularly within an aneurysm, often organized, adherent to wall |

| | |
|---|---|
| *Postoperative* | Right ventricular or septal patches (McCallum patch) |
| *Ductus arteriosus* | AP window location |
| *Left atrial myxoma* | Attached to septum, may be pedunculated |

## 70. ENLARGED ASCENDING AORTA

| | |
|---|---|
| **Hypertension** | Usually associated atherosclerotic calcification |
| **Aortic aneurysm** | Atherosclerotic; mycotic; Marfan syndrome—ascending aortic aneurysm ("tulip bulb" configuration) and dissection are common |
| **Aortic stenosis** | Valve calcification may be seen |
| Aortic insufficiency | Left ventricular enlargement occurs when advanced |
| Coarctation | Most commonly postductal narrowing and often collateral vessels, usually due to concomitant bicuspid aortic valve |
| *Uncommon* | Patent ductus arteriosus, syphilitic aortitis |

## 71. ENLARGED PULMONARY ARTERIES

**Pulmonary artery hypertension**
Decreased peripheral vessel caliber; severe lung disease—fibrosis, emphysema, pneumoconiosis, sarcoidosis; vasculitis; emboli—blood, tumor, fat; primary—idiopathic in young women; Eisenmenger

**Left-to-right shunt**
ASD, VSD, PDA, endocardial cushion defect, anomalous pulmonary venous return

**Pulmonary venous hypertension**
Mild PA enlargement; CHF, fluid overload, renal failure, LA obstruction—myxoma, constrictive pericarditis, mitral insufficiency, or stenosis; TAPVR below the diaphragm (cyanotic)

High-output heart disease
Anemia, sickle cell, fluid overload, AV fistulas, polycythemia vera, pregnancy, thyrotoxicosis

| | |
|---|---|
| *Pulmonary valve stenosis* | Enlarged main and left PA, normal right |
| *Behçet disease* | Rare vasculitis; pulmonary hemorrhage, thrombosis, and PA aneurysms are uncommon |
| *Idiopathic dilatation* | May be normal in young adult |
| *Hypoventilation* | Venoconstrictive hypertension, high altitude, neuromuscular disorder, obesity, tracheal obstruction, sleep apnea |

## 72. ENLARGED SUPERIOR VENA CAVA

| | |
|---|---|
| **Congestive heart failure** | Cardiomegaly, edema, pleural effusions |
| Cardiac tamponade | Constrictive pericarditis, pericardial effusion |
| Idiopathic | |
| *Anomalous pulmonary venous return* | Anomalous vein in lung is seen draining to mediastinum |

### Obstruction

| | |
|---|---|
| **Central bronchogenic carcinoma** | Small cell, squamous cell |
| Central venous catheter | Bland thrombus |
| Fibrosing mediastinitis | Idiopathic; granulomatous inflammation—histoplasmosis, calcified nodes often present |
| *Radiation therapy* | Fibrosis |

# PERITONEUM, MESENTERY, AND RETROPERITONEUM

## 73. PNEUMOPERITONEUM

| | |
|---|---|
| **Perforated bowel or stomach** | Ulcer, diverticulitis, obstruction, trauma, endoscopy, cancer, appendicitis |
| **Recent surgery** | Generally resolves within 1 week |
| Paracentesis | Ascites |
| Peritoneal dialysis | May include hydropneumoperitoneum |
| *Pneumothorax* | Pleuroperitoneal communication |
| *Transvaginal introduction* | Rare and inconsequential |

# 74. ASCITES

| | |
|---|---|
| **Cirrhosis** | Nodular liver surface, findings of portal hypertension |
| **Carcinomatosis** | Peritoneal metastases from ovarian or gastrointestinal primary |
| CHF | Distended IVC/hepatic veins, nutmeg liver with mottled enhancement |
| Renal failure | Small, atrophic kidneys |
| Hypoproteinemia | Nephrotic syndrome |
| Constrictive pericarditis | Distended IVC/hepatic veins, nutmeg liver with mottled enhancement, thickened or calcified pericardium |
| Peritonitis | Ascites, adenitis, peritoneal enhancement |
| Tuberculosis | Exudative ascites, adenopathy (low attenuation), mesenteric masses |
| IVC or portal vein obstruction | Enlarged azygous and other collaterals, cavernous transformation of portal vein |

| | |
|---|---|
| *Pancreatitis* | Idiopathic, alcohol, cholelithiasis, post-ERCP, viral; low-attenuation, peripancreatic soft tissue; potential for phlegmon, pseudocyst, abscess, hemorrhage, necrosis, pseudoaneurysm |
| *Appendicitis* | CT >95% sensitive and specific; ascites, soft tissue stranding, abscess, 25% appendicolith |
| *Lymphoma* | Can mimic carcinomatosis, may include mesenteric and retroperitoneal adenopathy |
| *Disrupted or obstructed lymphatics* | Trauma, surgery, tumor, filariasis |
| *Meig syndrome* | Benign ovarian fibroma with hydrothorax, generally on right |
| *Mimic* | Cyst, bowel loop, lymphocele, biloma, urinoma, pseudocyst, hematoma |

## 75. ABDOMINAL ABSCESS

| | |
|---|---|
| **Postoperative** | Soft tissue stranding, pneumoperitoneum |
| **Crohn disease** | 80% of patients have small bowel involvement, 50% with small bowel and colonic disease |
| **Appendicitis** | CT >95% sensitive and specific; ascites, soft tissue stranding, abscess, 25% appendicolith |
| **Diverticulitis** | 80% diverticular disease in sigmoid; pericolonic stranding, abscess, wall thickening; may be right-sided |
| **Pancreatitis** | Idiopathic, alcohol, cholelithiasis, post-ERCP, viral; abscess <10% |
| Perforated carcinoma | Generally colonic |
| Tuboovarian | STD-related, usually in cul-de-sac/adnexa; complex, cystic mass with soft tissue stranding |

| | |
|---|---|
| Ischemic colitis | Pericolonic stranding, wall thickening, pneumatosis, pneumoperitoneum |
| Tuberculosis | Adenopathy (low attenuation), exudative ascites, mesenteric masses, may cause small bowel obstruction |
| Pyelonephritis | Heterogeneous renal enhancement, perinephric stranding |

## 76. PERITONEAL LESION

| | |
|---|---|
| **Peritoneal metastases** | Ovarian and gastrointestinal primaries, masses and soft tissue infiltration, ascites |
| **Ascites** | Layers dependently and along mesentery |
| **Abscess** | Thick-walled and complex cystic lesion |
| Peritonitis | Ascites, adenitis, peritoneal enhancement |
| Lymphoma | Can mimic carcinomatosis; mesenteric and retroperitoneal adenopathy |
| Pancreatic pseudocyst | Most within or adjacent to gland, evaluate for other findings of pancreatitis (peritoneal location is uncommon) |
| Tuberculosis | Adenopathy (low attenuation), exudative ascites, mesenteric masses, may cause small bowel obstruction |

| | |
|---|---|
| Endometriosis | May have cyclic pain, often recurs, can seed laparoscopic port |
| Desmoid | Benign, infiltrative fibrous tumor associated with Gardner syndrome and pregnancy |
| Pseudomyxoma peritonei | Low-attenuation masses that may scallop parenchymal organ margins, mucocele/mucinous tumor origin |
| Mesothelioma | Associated with asbestos exposure, usually in men; mesenteric nodules and thickening, minimal ascites |
| Mesenteric cyst | Water attenuation |

## 77. MESENTERIC MASS

| | |
|---|---|
| **Lymphadenopathy** | Multiple soft tissue nodules |
| **Lymphoma** | Can mimic carcinomatosis, mesenteric and retroperitoneal adenopathy |
| Hematoma | Trauma, surgery, coagulopathy |
| Panniculitis | Inflammation with stranding, potential fat necrosis |
| Carcinoid | Desmoplastic mesenteric mass, often with calcification, may thicken small bowel due to venous congestion |
| Metastases | Ovarian and gastrointestinal primaries |
| Mesothelioma | Associated with asbestos exposure, usually in men; mesenteric nodules and thickening, minimal ascites |

| | |
|---|---|
| Tuberculosis | Adenopathy (low attenuation), exudative ascites, mesenteric masses, may cause small bowel obstruction |
| Leiomyosarcoma | Large, heterogeneous soft tissue mass, may arise from IVC; metastases to liver, lung, peritoneum |
| Malignant fibrous histiocytoma | Common retroperitoneal malignancy; complex, large, and infiltrating mass |
| Stromal tumor | Neurofibroma, leiomyoma, lipoma |
| Pseudocyst | Most within or adjacent to gland, evaluate for other findings of pancreatitis |
| Duplication cyst | Water attenuation |
| Teratoma | Variable soft tissue, fat, and calcific components |
| Lymphangioma | Multiloculated, infiltrating, complex cystic mass |
| *Desmoplastic small round cell tumor* | Children, multifocal soft tissue masses, ascites |

## 78. RETROPERITONEAL FIBROSIS

| | |
|---|---|
| **Idiopathic** | Most common (50%) |
| **Hemorrhage** | Aortic aneurysm, surgery, trauma |
| Lymphoma | Particularly nodular sclerosing Hodgkin |
| Drugs | Methysergide, ergotamine, hydralazine |
| Postoperative | AAA repair, lymph node dissection |
| Retroperitoneal metastases | Breast, colon |
| Radiation | Lymphoma, pelvic malignancies |
| Desmoplastic tumor | Carcinoid, usually mesenteric |
| Granulomatous infection | Tuberculosis, histoplasmosis |
| Inflammation | Pancreatitis, diverticulitis, Crohn disease |

# 79. RETROPERITONEAL MASS

| | |
|---|---|
| **Lymphoma** | Abundant adenopathy, confluent mass may encase aorta or other structures |
| **Hematoma** | Aortic aneurysm, trauma, coagulopathy, femoral puncture |
| **Adenopathy** | Testicular, cervical primaries among others |
| Abscess | Thick-walled, complex, and partially cystic mass |
| Liposarcoma | Heterogeneous, infiltrating mass containing macroscopic fat, most common retroperitoneal malignancy |
| Malignant fibrous histiocytoma | Common retroperitoneal malignancy |
| Pseudocyst | Most within or adjacent to gland, evaluate for other findings of pancreatitis |
| Lipoma | Uniform fat density |

| | |
|---|---|
| Lymphangioma | Multiloculated, infiltrating complex cystic mass, most frequent after surgery |
| Leiomyosarcoma | Large, heterogeneous soft tissue mass, may arise from IVC; metastases to liver, lung, peritoneum |

# LIVER

## 80. HEPATOMEGALY

**Fatty infiltration**    Obesity, alcohol, steroids, diabetes, chemotherapy, hyperalimentation

**Metastases**    Lung, breast, colon, many others; most common hepatic malignancy

### Primary tumors

**Hepatocellular carcinoma**    Focal, multinodular, or diffuse; 25% invade portal veins; cirrhosis, hemochromatosis, and glycogen storage diseases predispose

Hemangioma    Most common benign liver neoplasm, >5 cm "giant"

Adenoma    Young women, oral contraceptives and glycogen storage diseases predispose, can be multiple, may hemorrhage

Hepatoblastoma    Most frequent childhood hepatic malignancy

| | |
|---|---|
| *Hemangio-endothelioma* | Children; mixed-attenuation, enhancing tumor; may include enlarged hepatic artery/high-output CHF |
| *Angiosarcoma* | Thorotrast, arsenic, PVC predispose; aggressive and hypervascular |

## Hepatic congestion

| | |
|---|---|
| **Heart failure** | Distended IVC/hepatic veins, nutmeg liver with mottled enhancement |
| Constrictive pericarditis | Thick or calcified pericardium, distended IVC/hepatic veins, nutmeg liver with mottled enhancement |
| Tricuspid insufficiency or stenosis | Distended IVC/hepatic veins, nutmeg liver with mottled enhancement |
| Budd-Chiari syndrome | No contrast enhancement of hepatic veins, mottled enhancement, ascites |
| Veno-occlusive disease | Particularly following bone marrow transplantation |

## Other diseases

| | |
|---|---|
| **Cirrhosis** | Generally right lobe atrophy with caudate/left lobe enlargement |
| Hepatitis A, B, C | Bacterial, viral, serum |
| Hemochromatosis | Increased attenuation, increased risk of HCC |
| Abscess | Bacterial, amebic, fungal |
| Storage diseases | Niemann-Pick—sphingolipidosis<br>Von Gierke—glycogen storage disease with increased risk of HCC/adenomas<br>Gaucher—glucocerebrosidase deficiency |
| Chronic granulomatous disease of childhood | Inherited immunodeficiency with PML dysfunction causing purulent infections, abscesses, adenitis |
| Lymphoma | Secondary lymphomatous involvement of liver in >50% of Hodgkin/NHL, but seldom depicted on imaging |
| Myeloproliferative disease | Myelofibrosis, polycythemia vera |

| | |
|---|---|
| Mononucleosis | Epstein-Barr virus |
| Riedel lobe | Large inferior extent of the posterior segment of the right hepatic lobe |
| *Sarcoidosis* | Half of all sarcoid patients have hepatomegaly, focal granulomas possible |
| *Schistosomiasis* | Periportal fibrosis and calcified septations |
| *Extramedullary hematopoiesis* | Splenomegaly, expanded marrow, other hematopoietic sites (posterior mediastinum) |
| *Uncommon* | Polycystic disease—multiple cysts; Wilson disease—copper accumulation, increased hepatic attenuation; amyloidosis—generally decreased hepatic attenuation and other organ involvement; malaria; tuberculosis—may include focal lesions and adenopathy; histoplasmosis |

# 81. LOW-DENSITY LIVER PRECONTRAST

| | |
|---|---|
| **Fatty liver** | Diffuse, geographic, focal, multinodular |

## Hepatic congestion

| | |
|---|---|
| Heart failure | Distended IVC/hepatic veins, nutmeg liver with mottled enhancement |
| Tricuspid stenosis/insufficiency | Distended IVC/hepatic veins, nutmeg liver with mottled enhancement |
| Constrictive pericarditis | Thick or calcified pericardium, distended IVC/hepatic veins, nutmeg liver with mottled enhancement |
| Budd-Chiari | Enlarged liver with ascites, no hepatic vein enhancement, collaterals, high-attenuation caudate |

## Other lesions

| | |
|---|---|
| Diffuse metastases | Lung, breast, colon, many others; most common hepatic malignancy |

| | |
|---|---|
| Storage diseases | Niemann-Pick—sphingolipidosis<br>Von Gierke—glycogen storage disease with increased risk of HCC/adenomas<br>Gaucher—glucocerebrosidase deficiency |
| *Amyloidosis* | Generally decreased hepatic attenuation and other organ involvement |

## 82. FATTY LIVER

| | |
|---|---|
| **Obesity** | Fat deposition elsewhere |
| **Steroids** | Cushing syndrome as well |
| **Alcohol** | Cytotoxic agent |
| Cirrhosis | Early finding with small right hepatic lobe, enlarged caudate/left lobe, signs of portal hypertension |
| Cystic fibrosis | Pancreatic fatty replacement, may lead to biliary cirrhosis |
| Diabetes mellitus | Vascular calcifications |
| Chemotherapy | Cytotoxic agents |
| Hyperalimentation | Intravenous |
| Hyperlipidemia | Atherosclerotic disease |
| Storage diseases | Niemann-Pick—sphingolipidosis
Von Gierke—glycogen storage disease with increased risk of HCC/adenomas
Gaucher—glucocerebrosidase deficiency |

# 83. HIGH-DENSITY LIVER PRECONTRAST

| | |
|---|---|
| Primary hemochromatosis | Autosomal recessive, increased risk of HCC; diabetes, bronze skin, cardiomyopathy |
| Hemosiderosis | Numerous blood transfusions |
| Amiodarone | Iodine deposition, often with basilar pulmonary infiltrates or fibrosis, normal spleen |
| Storage diseases | More often low-density |
| Wilson disease | Autosomal recessive, copper deposition |
| *Gold* | Treatment of rheumatoid arthritis |
| *Thorotrast* | Alpha-emitting contrast agent no longer used, angiosarcoma predisposition |

## 84. HEPATIC CALCIFICATIONS

| | |
|---|---|
| **Old healed granulomatous disease** | Tuberculosis, histoplasmosis, coccidiomycosis |
| **Metastases** | Colon, breast, stomach, ovarian, melanoma, osteosarcoma, thyroid, teratoma, chondrosarcoma primaries; also following radiation or chemotherapy |

### Primary tumors

| | |
|---|---|
| Hepatocellular carcinoma | Occasional calcification |
| Fibrolamellar carcinoma | 30% calcify; uncommon form of HCC, younger patients, no cirrhosis, less aggressive |
| Hemangioma | Phleboliths are uncommon, low-attenuation lesion with peripheral, puddling enhancement which gradually fills in with contrast |
| Hemangio-endothelioma | Children; enhancing tumor may have enlarged hepatic artery/high-output CHF |

| | |
|---|---|
| Hepatoblastoma | Most frequent childhood hepatic malignancy |
| *Cholangio-carcinoma* | Central location most common with dilated bile ducts, potential delayed enhancement |

## Other lesions

| | |
|---|---|
| Hydatid cyst | *Echinococcus granulosus,* 25% calcify |
| Chronic abscess | Pyogenic, amebic, fungal |
| Calcified gallbladder | Porcelain gallbladder, associated with gallbladder cancer |
| Old hematoma | Posttraumatic, underlying lesion (adenoma) |
| Regenerating nodules | Rarely calcify, usually high attenuation on noncontrast CT |
| Chronic granulomatous disease of childhood | Inherited immunodeficiency with PML dysfunction causing purulent infections, abscesses, adenitis |
| Mimic | Lipoidal embolization (focal); hemochromatosis, hemosiderosis, Thorotrast (diffuse) |

## 85. LIVER LESION

**Cyst**  2% of all patients; increased in polycystic liver/kidney disease, VHL

**Focal fat**  Pericholecystic, periligamentous, perihilar; geographic low attenuation

### Malignant tumors

**Metastases**  Lung, breast, colon, many others; most common hepatic malignancy

**Hepatocellular carcinoma**  Multinodular, focal, or diffuse; 25% invade portal veins; cirrhosis, hemochromatosis, and glycogen storage diseases predispose

Cholangio-carcinoma  Central most common with dilated bile ducts, potential delayed enhancement

Fibrolamellar carcinoma  Uncommon form of HCC, younger patients, no cirrhosis, less aggressive

| | |
|---|---|
| Lymphoma | Secondary lymphomatous involvement in >50% of Hodgkin/NHL |
| Hepatoblastoma | Most common childhood hepatic malignancy, increased AFP and hormones |
| *Angiosarcoma* | Thorotrast, arsenic, PVC predispose; aggressive and hypervascular |
| *Kaposi sarcoma* | AIDS, often hypervascular |
| *Hemangio-endothelioma* | Children; enhancing tumor; may have enlarged hepatic artery/high-output CHF |

## Benign tumors

| | |
|---|---|
| **Hemangioma** | Most common liver neoplasm, low-attenuation lesion with peripheral, puddling enhancement which gradually fills in with contrast |
| Focal nodular hyperplasia | <20% multiple, peripheral, hypervascular, central scar |
| Regenerating nodule | Cirrhosis, usually high attenuation precontrast |

| | |
|---|---|
| Adenoma | May hemorrhage, young women, oral contraceptives and glycogen storage diseases predispose |
| Biliary cystadenoma | Multiloculated, cystic mass; excised and difficult to distinguish from carcinoma |

## Other lesions

| | |
|---|---|
| Abscess | Pyogenic, amebic, fungal |
| Hematoma | Posttraumatic, underlying lesion (adenoma) |
| *Hamartoma* | Partially cystic with hypervascular solid components, associated with polycystic liver disease |

## 86. MULTIPLE LIVER LESIONS

| | |
|---|---|
| **Metastases** | Lung, breast, colon, many others; most common hepatic malignancy |
| **Cysts** | Idiopathic, also 60% of patients with APCKD |
| **Hemangiomas** | Low-attenuation lesions with peripheral, puddling enhancement which gradually fills in with contrast |
| Hepatocellular carcinoma | Multinodular, focal, or diffuse; 25% invade portal veins; cirrhosis, hemochromatosis, and glycogen storage disease predispose |
| Focal nodular hyperplasia | <20% multiple, peripheral, hypervascular, central scar |
| Regenerating nodules | Usually high attenuation on noncontrast CT |
| Caroli disease | Multiple cystic masses and dilated bile ducts, 80% have medullary sponge kidney |
| *Adenomatosis* | Distinct from multiple adenomas |

## 87. LOW-DENSITY LIVER LESION PRECONTRAST

| | |
|---|---|
| **Cyst** | Water attenuation, no enhancement, imperceptible wall, 2% of all patients; increased in polycystic liver disease, polycystic kidney disease, VHL |
| **Focal fatty infiltration** | Periligamentous, pericholecystic, perihilar; geographic low attenuation |

### Malignant tumors

| | |
|---|---|
| **Metastases** | Lung, breast, colon, many others; most common hepatic malignancy |
| Hepatocellular carcinoma | Multinodular, focal, or diffuse; 25% invade portal veins; cirrhosis, hemochromatosis, and glycogen storage diseases predispose |
| Cholangio-carcinoma | Central most common with dilated bile ducts, potential delayed enhancement |

| | |
|---|---|
| Lymphoma | Secondary lymphomatous involvement in >50% of Hodgkin/NHL |

**Benign tumors**

| | |
|---|---|
| **Hemangioma** | Low-attenuation lesion with peripheral, puddling enhancement which gradually fills in with contrast |
| Focal nodular hyperplasia | <20% multiple, peripheral, hypervascular, central scar |
| Adenoma | Hypervascular with capsule; may hemorrhage; young women; oral contraceptives and glycogen storage diseases predispose |

**Abscesses**

| | |
|---|---|
| Pyogenic | Complex, cystic lesions with rim enhancement; may cluster; few with gas |
| Amebic | *Entamoeba histolytica,* majority in right hepatic lobe, generally solitary |
| Fungal | *Candida, Cryptococcus;* numerous low-attenuation microabscesses |

| | |
|---|---|
| Parasitic | Hydatid disease, schistosomiasis |

**Other lesions**

| | |
|---|---|
| Hematoma | Posttraumatic, underlying lesion (adenoma) |
| Biloma | Posttraumatic, intervention |
| Infarct | Uncommon due to dual blood supply |
| Radiation therapy | Leads to local fatty replacement, geographic margins corresponding to port |

## 88. LOW-DENSITY LIVER LESION POSTCONTRAST

### Tumors

| | |
|---|---|
| **Metastases** | Lung, breast, colon, many others; most common hepatic malignancy |
| Giant hemangioma | >5-cm, low-attenuation lesion with peripheral, puddling enhancement which gradually fills in with contrast |
| Cystic masses | Biliary cystadenoma/cystadenocarcinoma, Caroli disease, lymphangioma |
| Primary tumor | Cholangiocarcinoma with late enhancement |
| Regenerating nodules | Hyperdense precontrast, cirrhotic liver |

### Other lesions

| | |
|---|---|
| **Cyst** | Water attenuation, no enhancement, imperceptible wall, 2% of all patients; increased in polycystic liver disease, polycystic kidney disease, VHL |

| | |
|---|---|
| **Focal fatty infiltration** | Periligamentous, pericholecystic, perihilar; geographic |
| Abscess | Complex, thick walls, right lobe predilection |
| Hematoma | Posttraumatic, underlying lesion (adenoma) |

## 89. LIVER CYST

| | |
|---|---|
| **Epithelial** | Water attenuation, no enhancement, imperceptible wall, 2% of all patients |
| **Traumatic** | Hematoma or biloma |
| **Adult polycystic kidney disease** | Up to 40% of APCKD patients |
| **Cystic metastasis** | Ovarian, gastric primaries |
| Abscess | Complex, thick walls, right lobe predilection for amebic abscesses |
| Von Hippel-Lindau | Renal cysts, renal cell carcinoma, pheochromocytomas and neurocutaneous manifestations |
| Biliary cystadenoma or cystadenocarcinoma | Multiloculated, cystic mass; excised and difficult to distinguish benign from malignant |
| Choledochal cyst | RUQ pain, mass, jaundice |
| Hydatid disease | *Echinococcus granulosus,* daughter cysts, calcification, fluid-fluid levels |

| | |
|---|---|
| Caroli disease | Multiple cystic masses and dilated bile ducts, 80% have medullary sponge kidney |
| *Lymphangioma* | Mesenchymal hamartoma, generally in children, complex cystic mass/may have solid elements |

# 90. HYPERVASCULAR LIVER LESION

## Malignant tumors

**Hepatocellular carcinoma**  Less commonly hypervascular; multinodular, focal, or diffuse; 25% invade portal veins; cirrhosis, hemochromatosis, and glycogen storage diseases predispose

**Vascular metastases**  Carcinoid, melanoma, islet cell, breast, sarcoma

*Hemangio-endothelioma*  Children; enhancing tumor; may have enlarged hepatic artery/high-output CHF

*Angiosarcoma*  Thorotrast, arsenic, PVC predisposes

## Benign tumors

**Hemangioma**  Low-attenuation lesion with peripheral, puddling enhancement which gradually fills in with contrast

Adenoma  Capsule, may hemorrhage, young women, oral contraceptives predispose

| | |
|---|---|
| Focal nodular hyperplasia | Peripheral, hypervascular, asymptomatic, central scar |
| Regenerating nodules | Hyperdense precontrast, cirrhotic liver |

**Other lesions**

| | |
|---|---|
| **Focal fatty-sparing** | Simulates enhancing mass, background of hepatic low attenuation |
| Vascular phenomena | SVC obstruction (enhancement adjacent to falciform), Budd-Chiari (enhancement in caudate), transient hepatic attenuation difference (THAD) |
| Arteriovenous malformation | Congenital or following intervention |
| *Hepatic artery aneurysm* | Trauma or inflammation |

## 91. LIVER LESION WITH CENTRAL SCAR

**Focal nodular hyperplasia** — Central scar high signal on T2 MR, <20% multiple, peripheral, hypervascular

Fibrolamellar hepatocellular carcinoma — Central scar low signal on T2 MR, uncommon form of HCC, younger patients, no cirrhosis, less aggressive

Hemangioma — Low-attenuation lesion with peripheral puddling enhancement which gradually fills in with contrast

Adenoma — Hypervascular with capsule, may hemorrhage, young women, oral contraceptives and glycogen storage diseases predispose

## 92. PORTAL VENOUS GAS

| | |
|---|---|
| **Mesenteric ischemia, necrosis, or infarction** | Ominous finding |
| **Pneumobilia (mimic)** | Central |
| Bowel obstruction | Does not necessitate infarction |
| Necrotizing enterocolitis | Children; may resolve, complication of bowel strictures |
| Diverticulitis, intraabdominal abscess | Low-density lesion with thick, enhancing margin |
| Inflammatory bowel disease | Following barium enema or colonoscopy |
| Recent bowel surgery | Intraabdominal stranding, fluid |
| Toxic megacolon | 10% of ulcerative colitis patients; Crohn disease, CMV, ischemia, pseudomembranous colitis, amebiasis |

# GALLBLADDER AND BILE DUCTS

## 93. ENLARGED GALLBLADDER

| | |
|---|---|
| **Fasting or hyper-alimentation** | Distention with normal wall |
| **Cholelithiasis or obstructing stone** | Distention often with thickened wall, pericholecystic stranding, Murphy sign |
| Pancreatitis | Pancreatic edema, gallbladder wall may be thickened |
| Pancreatic head mass | Adenocarcinoma, dilated biliary tree |
| Diabetes | |
| Drugs | Narcotics, anticholinergics |
| AIDS | Cholangiopathy with thickened biliary epithelium, *Cryptosporidium*/CMV |

## 94. DILATED COMMON BILE DUCT WITHOUT OBSTRUCTION

| | |
|---|---|
| **Aging** | 6 mm at 60 years, 1-mm increase each additional decade |
| **Prior biliary surgery** | Including cholecystectomy |
| Recent stone passage | Ampullary edema, adjacent inflammation |
| Choledochal cyst | Type I with fusiform CBD dilatation |

## 95. INTRAHEPATIC BILIARY DILATATION

| | |
|---|---|
| **Obstructing stone** | CBD stone or intrahepatic pigmented stone |
| **Pancreatic head mass** | Adenocarcinoma with painless jaundice |
| **Stricture** | Prior surgery, inflammation, idiopathic |
| **Sclerosing cholangitis** | Beaded and thickened intra/extrahepatic ducts; increased rate with ulcerative colitis, Crohn disease, and retroperitoneal fibrosis |
| Caroli disease | Multiple cystic masses and dilated bile ducts, 80% have medullary sponge kidney |
| Periportal edema (mimic) | On both sides of central portal veins |
| Periportal adenopathy | Hepatic, pancreatic, gastric, lymphomatous primaries |
| Infectious cholangitis | Bacterial, parasitic, viral (HIV) |

| | |
|---|---|
| Hepatic fibrosis | Cholestasis, may be in conjunction with polycystic disease |

# 96. DIFFUSE GALLBLADDER WALL THICKENING

**Incomplete distention**

| | |
|---|---|
| **Ascites** | Renal failure, cirrhosis, hypoalbuminemia, heart failure |
| **Cholecystitis** | Acute or chronic, cholelithiasis, pericholecystic stranding, Murphy sign |
| **Adjacent inflammation** | Hepatitis, pancreatitis, peptic ulcer |
| Gallbladder carcinoma | Wall thickening or discrete mass; cholelithiasis and chronic cholecystitis generally present, may invade liver |
| AIDS | Cholangiopathy with thickened biliary epithelium; *Cryptosporidium,* cytomegalovirus, AIDS virus itself |
| Adenomyomatosis | Hyperplastic overgrowth of wall, focal or diffuse, Rokitansky-Aschoff sinuses |

## 97. FOCAL GALLBLADDER WALL THICKENING

| | |
|---|---|
| **Inflammatory polyp** | <1-cm lesion can be followed, >1-cm lesion excised for cancer risk |
| **Adenomyomatosis** | Hyperplastic overgrowth of wall, focal or diffuse, Rokitansky-Aschoff sinuses |
| **Gallbladder carcinoma** | Wall thickening or discrete mass; cholelithiasis and chronic cholecystitis generally present, may invade liver |
| **Adherent stone/sludge** | Can attempt to reposition patient, 25% of stones isodense to bile |
| Metastasis | Melanoma |
| Benign tumor | Adenoma, papilloma, carcinoid |
| Varices | Tubular and enhancing |
| Ectopic mucosa | Uncommon |

## 98. HIGH-ATTENUATION BILE

| | |
|---|---|
| **Vicarious excretion of contrast** | Renal failure, recent ERCP; a small percentage of normal individuals will demonstrate contrast in bile on delayed images |
| **Cholelithiasis** | 25% of stones are isodense to bile |
| Milk of calcium | Layers dependently with fluid-fluid level |
| Hematobilia | Posttraumatic |

## 99. PNEUMOBILIA

| | |
|---|---|
| **Sphincterotomy** | Often mild pancreatitis following ERCP |
| **Recent gallstone passage** | Cholelithiasis, duct dilatation |
| Cholecystoenterostomy or choledochoenterostomy | Whipple procedure |
| Emphysematous cholecystitis | Diabetics |
| Trauma | Generally penetrating |
| Gallstone ileus | SBO, ectopic gallstone usually at terminal ileum, pneumobilia (Rigler triad) |
| Enteric fistula | Cholecystitis, perforated ulcer, or cancer |

# SPLEEN

## 100. SMALL SPLEEN

| | |
|---|---|
| **Splenule** | 10 to 30% of normal patients have splenule in addition to normal spleen |
| Trauma | Splenic rupture/fragmentation |
| Infarction | Sickle cell disease, increased attenuation |
| Polysplenia | Multiple small splenules, often bilateral |
| Uncommon | Hypoplasia, radiation, atrophy |

## 101. SPLENOMEGALY (>13-cm cephalocaudal span)

### Masses

| | |
|---|---|
| **Lymphoma** | Most common primary splenic malignancy, nodules or diffuse infiltration |
| Leukemia | Particularly CML |
| Cyst | Posttraumatic, hydatid, epithelial |
| Metastases | Melanoma, breast, lung, ovary, colon |

### Other causes

| | |
|---|---|
| **Congestion** | CHF, portal hypertension/thrombosis, cirrhosis |
| **Hemolytic anemia** | Spherocytosis, hemoglobinopathies |
| **Infection** | Mononucleosis, HIV/AIDS, candidiasis, histoplasmosis, malaria |
| Hematoma | Trauma |
| Sarcoid | Up to 30% of patients have splenomegaly |

| | |
|---|---|
| Extramedullary hematopoiesis | Myelofibrosis, polycythemia vera |
| Storage diseases | Niemann-Pick—sphingolipidosis<br>Von Gierke—glycogen storage disease<br>Gaucher—glucocerebrosidase deficiency |
| Chronic granulomatous disease of childhood | Inherited immunodeficiency with PML dysfunction causing purulent infections, abscesses, adenitis |
| Collagen vascular disease | Lupus |
| *Amyloidosis* | Hypodense spleen |

## 102. SPLENIC LESION

### Benign tumors

**Hemangioma** — Most common benign splenic tumor, speckled calcifications uncommon, peripheral contrast wash-in

Lymphangioma — Multiloculated cystic lesion, frequent calcification

Hamartoma — Low attenuation

### Malignant tumors

**Lymphoma** — Most common primary splenic malignancy, nodules or diffuse infiltration

Leukemia — Usually CML

Metastases — Melanoma, breast, ovary, lung, colon

*Angiosarcoma and rare neoplasms* — Hypervascular, poor prognosis

### Other lesions

**Cyst** — Posttraumatic, hydatid, epithelial, pseudocyst from pancreatitis

| | |
|---|---|
| **Infarct** | Peripheral, other organs may be involved |
| **Abscess** | Pyogenic, candidal, *Pneumocystis carinii* |
| **Hematoma** | Posttraumatic |
| Sarcoid | 15% of patients have hypodense granulomata |
| Inflammatory pseudotumor | Inflammatory cell infiltrate, heterogeneous and hypodense mass |
| *Peliosis* | Blood-filled spaces in reticuloendothelial system, hypodense lesions |
| *Arteriovenous malformation* | Can contain phleboliths, large lesion can show enlarged splenic artery/vein |

## 103. SPLENIC CYST

| | |
|---|---|
| **Posttraumatic cyst** | 80% of splenic cysts |
| **Congenital/ epithelial cyst** | <20% of splenic cysts |
| **Abscess** | Pyogenic, candidal, *Pneumocystis carinii* |
| Hemangioma | Most common benign splenic tumor, peripheral contrast wash-in |
| Lymphangioma | Multiloculated cystic lesion, frequent calcification |
| *Hydatid cyst* | *Echinococcus granulosus* |
| *Dissecting pancreatic pseudocyst* | Findings of acute or chronic pancreatitis |

## 104. SPLENIC CALCIFICATIONS

| | |
|---|---|
| **Atherosclerotic splenic artery** | Possible aneurysm/pseudoaneurysm |
| **Healed granulomatous disease** | Tuberculosis, histoplasmosis |
| **Sickle cell disease** | Microscopic calcium deposition, diffusely increased attenuation |
| Cyst with rim calcification | Posttraumatic, hydatid, epithelial |
| Healed hematoma | Trauma, coagulopathy |
| Hemangioma | Phleboliths |
| Increased density (mimic) | Sickle cell disease, hemochromatosis, Thorotrast |
| *Pneumocystis carinii* | Multiple small round foci |
| Infarction | Marginated, peripheral; other organs (kidneys) may be involved |
| Abscess | Pyogenic, candidal, *Pneumocystis carinii* |

# PANCREAS

## 105. PANCREATIC FATTY CHANGE

| | |
|---|---|
| **Aging** | Global glandular atrophy |
| **Cystic fibrosis** | Often with no discernible pancreatic tissue |
| Obesity | Fat deposition elsewhere |
| Steroids | Cushing syndrome as well |
| Malnutrition | Diminished fat elsewhere |
| *Schwachman-Diamond syndrome* | Congenital pancreatic exocrine insufficiency |

# 106. PANCREATIC CALCIFICATION

| | |
|---|---|
| **Chronic pancreatitis** | Alcoholic, hereditary, or biliary; intraductal calcifications |
| **Vascular calcifications** | Atherosclerotic disease elsewhere |

## Tumors

| | |
|---|---|
| Adenocarcinoma | <2% calcify |
| Islet cell (pancreatic endocrine) tumor | 20% calcify |
| Microcystic cystadenoma | Sunburst calcifications, benign, serous fluid, elderly patients |
| Metastases | Mucinous gastrointestinal primaries |
| Hemangioma | Phleboliths |

## Other lesions

| | |
|---|---|
| Pseudocyst | Calcification in wall, chronic |
| Prior hematoma | Trauma, coagulopathy |
| Cystic fibrosis | Fatty replacement, biliary cirrhosis |

| | |
|---|---|
| Hemochromatosis | Pancreatic involvement gives endocrine insufficiency and "bronze diabetes" |

## 107. PANCREATIC CYST

**Pseudocyst** — Develops in >30% of acute pancreatitis, thick wall, takes >4 weeks to develop

**Adult polycystic kidney disease** — 10% of APCKD patients, VHL with pancreatic cysts more commonly

Congenital/epithelial — Uncommon

### Tumor

Microcystic adenoma — Serous fluid, generally small cysts, sunburst calcifications, elderly patients/VHL

Macrocystic adenoma — Mucinous, malignant evolution, large and multiloculated

Solid and papillary neoplasm — Low-grade malignancy of young women, variably cystic

## 108. PANCREATIC MASS

### Malignant tumors

**Adenocarcinoma**  <2% calcify; 50% with biliary dilatation; obliterated peripancreatic fat planes, adenopathy, hepatic metastases

Lymphoma  Peripancreatic adenopathy, large lesion, most are secondary tumors

Metastases  Melanoma, renal cell, breast, lung, stomach

Duct ectatic mucinous tumor  Dilated pancreatic duct with increased mucin production

Solid and papillary neoplasm  Low-grade malignancy of young women, variably cystic

*Acinar cell carcinoma*  Systemic fat necrosis due to lipase production

## Potentially malignant

| | |
|---|---|
| Islet cell (pancreatic endocrine) tumors | 70 to 80% hyperfunctional, hypervascular, 60% in body and tail, 20% calcify<br>Insulinoma—>60% of hyperfunctional, 90% benign, marked contrast enhancement, small, 10% multiple<br>Gastrinoma—20% of hyperfunctional; pancreatic head, duodenal or gastric wall; 60% malignant, 60% multiple<br>Nonfunctioning—large at presentation as clinically silent<br>Rare forms—often large because symptoms nonspecific; glucagonoma, somatostatinoma, VIPoma |
| Macrocystic adenoma | Mucinous, malignant evolution, large and multiloculated |

## Other lesions

| | |
|---|---|
| **Pseudocyst** | Develops in >30% of acute pancreatitis, takes >4 weeks to develop, thick capsule |
| Microcystic adenoma | Serous fluid, generally small cysts, sunburst calcifications, elderly patients/VHL |
| Mimic | Celiac axis adenopathy, adrenal mass, splenule |
| Focal pancreatitis | Adjacent inflammation, <10% with hemorrhage or necrosis; alcohol, viral, cholelithiasis, drug and familial associations |

## 109. HYPERVASCULAR PANCREATIC MASS

**Islet cell tumor** — Insulinoma, gastrinoma, nonhyperfunctioning

Microcystic adenoma — Serous fluid, generally small cysts, sunburst calcifications, elderly patients/VHL

Metastases — Renal cell, melanoma, carcinoid

Solid and papillary neoplasm — Low-grade malignancy of young women, variably cystic

Pseudoaneurysm — Postpancreatitis, hepatic or gastroduodenal arteries

# ADRENAL GLANDS

## 110. ADRENAL MASS

### Benign tumors

**Adenoma** — Low density (<10 to 18 HU) on noncontrast CT, Cushing and Conn syndromes

Myelolipoma — Macroscopic fat and bone marrow elements

Pheochromo-cytoma — 10% multiple, 10% bilateral, 10% extraadrenal, 10% pediatric, 10% malignant; associated with MEN IIA and B, NF, TS, and VHL

Ganglioneuroma — Mature, benign neural crest tumor; 10% in adrenal gland with most in posterior mediastinum

### Malignant tumors

**Metastases** — Lung, breast, renal cell

**Neuroblastoma** — Children and infants, 50% with calcification

Adrenocortical carcinoma — Large, partially necrotic mass; 50% functional—generally at low levels

| | |
|---|---|
| Lymphoma | Non-Hodgkin type, bilateral and preserve shape, adenopathy elsewhere and often renal involvement |

**Other lesions**

| | |
|---|---|
| **Hyperplasia** | Bilateral, possibly nodular; cushingoid features |
| Hemorrhage | Coagulopathy, severe stress, trauma, sepsis; may form pseudocyst |
| Granulomatous disease | Tuberculosis, histoplasmosis; may be cystic or calcified |
| Cyst | 45% epithelial, 40% pseudocysts generally from hemorrhage |
| Infection | Histoplasmosis, tuberculosis; bilateral enlargement early in course |
| Mimic | Pancreatic tail, fluid-filled bowel, renal apex, gastric diverticulum, collateral vessels (especially in patients with cirrhosis) |

# 111. ADRENAL CALCIFICATION

## Tumors

| | |
|---|---|
| **Neuroblastoma** | Speckled, 50% calcify |
| Adrenocortical carcinoma | Typically large mass, 30% calcify |
| Metastases | Mucinous primaries, posthemorrhage |
| Adenoma | Low density (<10 to 18 HU) on noncontrast CT, Cushing and Conn syndromes |
| Myelolipoma | Macroscopic fat and bone marrow elements |
| Pheochromocytoma | Eggshell calcification |
| Ganglioneuroma | Similar CT appearance to neuroblastoma |

## Other lesions

| | |
|---|---|
| **Prior hemorrhage** | Coagulopathy, trauma, sepsis, dehydration |
| Infection/abscess | Tuberculosis, histoplasmosis; late in course, patients may develop Addison disease |

| | |
|---|---|
| Waterhouse-Friderichsen syndrome | Meningococcal infection sequela |
| *Wolman disease* | Autosomal recessive lipidosis with hepatosplenomegaly, fatal |

# KIDNEYS

# 112. UNILATERAL SMALL KIDNEY
(atrophy or hypoplasia)

**Postobstructive atrophy** — Dilated collecting system and thin cortex

**Congenital hypoplasia** — Preserved shape, Ask-Upmark kidney with focal hypoplasia

**Ischemia** — Atherosclerosis, FMD, trauma to vascular pedicle

Radiation nephritis — Long-term sequelae

Infarction — Chronic, prior arterial or venous thrombosis

Multicystic dysplastic kidney — Hypoplastic form, numerous cysts, no cortical function/enhancement, may have peripheral calcification, 30% contralateral UPJ

Reflux nephropathy — Thinned cortex particularly over papillae, collecting system may be dilated

Postinfectious atrophy — Cortical scarring

Partial resection — Focal, geographic defect

# 113. BILATERAL SMALL KIDNEYS

| | |
|---|---|
| **Arteriosclerosis with ischemia** | Bilateral renal artery stenosis |
| **Chronic glomerulo-nephritis** | May include cortical nephrocalcinosis |
| Chronic papillary necrosis | Diabetes, sickle cell disease, analgesics |
| Bilateral obstructive atrophy | Dilated collecting system and thin cortex |
| Chronic pyelonephritis | Usually unilateral |
| Reflux nephropathy | Thinned cortex particularly over papillae, collecting system may be dilated |
| Diabetes | More commonly enlarged kidneys |
| Chronic hypertension | |

# 114. UNILATERAL LARGE KIDNEY

| | |
|---|---|
| **Compensatory hypertrophy** | Decreased contralateral renal function, postnephrectomy |
| **Obstruction or hydronephrosis** | Stone, tumor, stricture |
| **Primary tumor** | Renal cell carcinoma, Wilms tumor (may be seen at isthmus of horseshoe kidney) |
| **Acute pyelonephritis** | Delayed excretion, striated nephrogram, may have abscess |
| **Idiopathic** | Normal variant |
| Xanthogranulomatous pyelonephritis | Staghorn calculous, lipid-laden macrophage infiltration, *Proteus* infection |
| Duplex system | 20% bilateral |
| Cross-fused ectopia | >75% cross left to right |
| Polycystic kidney disease | >90% bilateral but may be asymmetric |
| Hematoma | Trauma, anticoagulation |

| | |
|---|---|
| Renal vein thrombosis | RCCA invasion, hypercoagulable state, sepsis, IVC clot extension |
| Acute infarction | Trauma, thromboembolic disease, vasculitis; small kidney over long term |
| Multicystic dysplastic kidney | Numerous cysts, no cortical function/enhancement, 30% contralateral UPJ obstruction |
| Multilocular cystic nephroma | Bimodal distribution (young boys and older women), complex cystic lesion |

## 115. BILATERAL LARGE KIDNEYS
(>13 cm in length)

| | |
|---|---|
| **Diabetes mellitus** | Vascular calcifications |
| **Normal variant** | |
| Acute papillary necrosis | Diabetes, sickle cell disease, phenacetin, postobstruction |
| Bilateral hydronephrosis | Retroperitoneal fibrosis, pelvic tumor, or radiation |
| AIDS nephropathy | High creatine is associated with poor outcome (50% death in 3 to 6 months) |
| Medullary sponge kidney | Usually normal or slight enlargement |
| Amyloidosis | Kidneys become small with chronic disease |
| Arterial infarction | Acute, diminished parenchymal enhancement, often with capsular collaterals |
| Renal vein thrombosis | Venous congestion, tumor or bland thrombus |
| Bilateral duplex system | 20% of cases, upper pole obstructs while lower pole refluxes |

Acute urate nephropathy

## Inflammation

| | |
|---|---|
| **Acute glomerulo-nephritis** | Streptococcal infection |
| Pyelonephritis | Delayed excretion, striated nephrogram, may contain abscess |
| Wegener granulomatosis | Focal glomerulonephritis, upper respiratory and sinus disease |
| Goodpasture disease | Autoimmune disease of young men; glomerulonephritis, pulmonary disease, and hemorrhage |
| Lupus, polyarteritis nodosa | Glomerulonephritis, microaneurysms |
| Acute interstitial nephritis | Drug reaction, eosinophilia |
| Acute tubular necrosis | Due to drugs or ischemia, edema enlarges kidneys, delayed or dense nephrogram |

| | |
|---|---|
| Acute cortical necrosis | Shock, dehydration, abruption; calcifies late in course |

## Masses

| | |
|---|---|
| **Polycystic kidney disease** | Lobulated from cysts |
| Lymphoma | NHL, diffuse involvement in medulla, multifocal masses (most common), lymphadenopathy |
| Leukemia | Diffuse renal involvement common |
| Metastases | Very common at autopsy; lung, breast, lymphoma, contralateral renal cell |
| Tuberous sclerosis | Multiple AMLs or cysts in >50% of TS patients |
| Multiple myeloma | Protein precipitation and amyloid deposition, small kidneys late |

## 116. RENAL CALCIFICATIONS

| | |
|---|---|
| **Atherosclerotic vessels** | Atherosclerotic disease elsewhere |
| **Nephrolithiasis** | 75% calcium oxalate ± calcium phosphate, all but matrix types dense on CT |
| **Renal cyst** | Thin wall is benign, thick wall prompts further evaluation or excision |
| Renal cell carcinoma | 15% have calcifications |
| **Medullary nephrocalcinosis** | |
| **Renal tubular acidosis** | Distal |
| **Hyperparathyroidism** | Hypercalcemia |
| **Medullary sponge kidney** | Calcifications in ectatic collecting ducts |
| Hypercalcemic states | Milk-alkali syndrome, idiopathic hypercalciuria, sarcoid, hypervitaminosis D |

| | |
|---|---|
| Cushing syndrome | 85% from pituitary adenomas |
| Paraneoplastic syndrome | Secondary hypercalcemia from diffuse metastases |
| Papillary necrosis | Necrotic papillae calcify; diabetes, sickle cell, phenacetin, others |

**Cortical nephrocalcinosis**

| | |
|---|---|
| **Chronic glomerulo-nephritis** | Poststreptococcal infection |
| Oxalosis | Primary hyperoxaluria |
| Acute cortical necrosis | Shock, dehydration, abruption |
| Alport syndrome | Nephrocalcinosis and nerve deafness, likely autosomal dominant |
| Chronic transplant rejection | Iliac fossa location |

## Other lesions

| | |
|---|---|
| Infection | Tuberculosis, abscess, xanthogranulomatous pyelonephritis, echinococcal cyst |
| Wilms tumor | Most common renal malignancy in children, 5% bilateral, necrosis is common, 30% involve renal vein |
| Multicystic dysplastic kidney | Numerous cysts, no cortical function/enhancement, may have peripheral calcification, 30% contralateral UPJ obstruction |
| Old hematoma | Trauma, coagulopathy, ESWL; typically peripheral |
| Furosemide therapy | Children |

## 117. HYDRONEPHROSIS

| | |
|---|---|
| **Ureteral obstruction** | Stone, tumor, extrinsic mass, retroperitoneal fibrosis, recent stone passage or instrumentation, posterior urethral valves, ectopic ureterocele, prune belly syndrome |
| **UPJ obstruction** | Congenital, crossing vessel |
| Reflux | Pediatric patients, ureteral diversion |
| Megacalicosis | Mostly men, club-shaped calyces with normal pelvis and infundibula, associated with megaureter, preserved function |
| *Megacystis-microcolon syndrome* | Rare lethal syndrome |
| Others | Diuresis, full bladder, bladder outlet obstruction |

## 118. RENAL MASS

| | |
|---|---|
| **Renal cyst** | 50% of patients over 50 years old |

**Malignant tumors**

| | |
|---|---|
| **Renal cell carcinoma** | >85% of adult renal malignancies, hypervascular with spread to nodes and renal vein |
| **Transitional cell carcinoma** | 5 to 10% of adult renal malignancies, poor enhancement, intraluminal extent, seeding of urothelium, "faceless kidney" |
| **Wilms** | Most common renal malignancy in children, 5% bilateral, necrosis is common, 30% involve renal vein, may occur at isthmus in a horseshoe kidney |
| Lymphoma/ leukemia | Diffuse, multifocal, or solitary mass; may engulf kidney |
| Metastases | Lung, breast, gastrointestinal, and melanoma primaries; common at autopsy |

| | |
|---|---|
| Squamous cell carcinoma | Avascular parenchymal mass, leukoplakia |
| *Clear cell sarcoma* | Children, bone metastases |
| *Rhabdoid tumor* | Children, associated CNS tumor, high mortality |
| *Sarcoma* | Usually from capsule; leiomyosarcoma, liposarcoma, PNET, and fibrosarcoma |

## Benign tumors

| | |
|---|---|
| **Angiomyolipoma** | Contains fat; multiple AMLs or cysts in >50% of tuberous sclerosis patients; only 20% of patients with AML have tuberous sclerosis |
| Multicystic dysplastic kidney | Numerous cysts, no cortical function/enhancement, may have peripheral calcification, 30% contralateral UPJ obstruction |
| Mesoblastic nephroma | Neonates, CT appearance like Wilms but no renal vein involvement |

| | |
|---|---|
| Multilocular cystic nephroma | Bimodal distribution (young boys/older women), complex cystic lesion, 50% calcify |
| Oncocytoma | Large tumor which may have central stellate scar in 30% |
| Reninoma | Juxtaglomerular apparatus origin, renin secretion produces hypertension |
| *Carcinoid* | Indistinguishable from RCCA |
| *Adenoma* | <2 to 3 cm, cannot differentiate benign from malignant |
| *Mesenchymal tumors* | Lipoma, hemangioma (young adult with intermittent hematuria), myoma, fibroma |

## Other lesions

| | |
|---|---|
| **Dromedary hump** | Splenic indentation creates focal protrusion on lateral border of left kidney |
| **Column of Bertin** | Pseudotumor of cortical hypertrophy into medulla, cortical attenuation |

| | |
|---|---|
| Abscess | Thick, irregular wall; associated perinephric inflammation; gas rare |
| Focal bacterial nephritis or infarct | Wedge-shaped region of low attenuation |
| Hematoma | Postprocedural, traumatic, coagulopathy |
| Xantho-granulomatous pyelonephritis | Staghorn calculus, lipid-laden macrophage infiltration, *Proteus* infection |
| Other childhood tumors | Nephroblastomatosis (Wilms association), congenital mesoblastic nephroma |
| Vascular | Renal artery aneurysm; arteriovenous malformation—congenital, postprocedural, traumatic |
| Tuberculoma | May lead to "putty kidney," calyceal amputation, urinary tract calcifications |

## 119. RENAL MASS WITH FAT

**Angiomyolipoma** — May hemorrhage; multiple AMLs or cysts in >50% of tuberous sclerosis patients; only 20% of patients with an AML have tuberous sclerosis

**Xantho-granulomatous pyelonephritis** — Lipid-laden macrophage infiltration, staghorn calculus, *Proteus* infection

Wilms tumor — Most common renal malignancy in children, 5% bilateral, necrosis is common, 30% involve renal vein

Renal cell carcinoma — May entrap perinephric or sinus fat, lipid necrosis

*Liposarcoma/lipoma* — Arise from capsule

*Teratoma* — Soft tissue, fat, and particularly calcification

## 120. RENAL CYSTS

**Cortical cysts (simple cysts)** — Water attenuation, imperceptible wall, no enhancement; hemorrhage/protein may cause hyperdense cyst

**Parapelvic cyst** — Adjacent to renal pelvis, rarely obstructs collecting system, can mimic hydronephrosis (normal calyces)

Calyceal diverticulum — Generally fills on delayed images

### Conditions associated with multiple cysts

**Adult polycystic disease** — Enlarged kidneys with numerous cysts, 60% with hepatic and 10% with pancreatic cysts

**Infantile polycystic disease** — Inverse severity of renal and hepatic disease

**Acquired cystic disease** — After long-term dialysis, small kidneys, predisposition to renal cell carcinoma

| | |
|---|---|
| Von Hippel-Lindau disease | >75% with renal cysts; 35% with RCCA which are often bilateral or multifocal |
| Medullary cystic disease | Tubulointerstitial fibrosis and small cysts, no calcifications, young patients |
| Medullary sponge kidney | Multiple small medullary cysts with calculi, bilateral in 70% |
| Tuberous sclerosis | 50% of TS patients have bilateral AMLs or cysts, cysts often early |
| Meckel-Gruber | Occipital encephalocele, polydactyly, autosomal recessive |
| Zellweger syndrome | Cerebrohepatorenal syndrome, brain dysgenesis, hepatomegaly, autosomal recessive |

**Cystic tumors**

| | |
|---|---|
| Cystic renal cell carcinoma | 5% of renal cells, usually thick wall or septations |
| Multilocular cystic nephroma | Bimodal distribution (young boys and older women), complex cystic lesion |

| | |
|---|---|
| Multicystic dysplastic kidney | Numerous cysts, no cortical function/enhancement, may have peripheral calcification, 30% contralateral UPJ obstruction |
| Angiomyolipoma | Fat simulating water attenuation, ROI distinguishes |
| Metastases | Lung, breast, melanoma, and gastrointestinal primaries |

## Other potentially cystic lesions

| | |
|---|---|
| Hydronephrosis | Dilated calyces connect to renal pelvis |
| Hematoma | Trauma, coagulopathy |
| Urinoma | Trauma or intervention |
| Vascular | Arteriovenous fistula, pseudoaneurysm as complication of intervention |
| *Hydatid* | May have calcification in wall |

## 121. PERINEPHRIC LESION

**Hematoma** — Trauma, tumor, anticoagulation, ESWL, AAA

**Perinephric abscess** — Pyelonephritis, tuberculosis

**Renal cell carcinoma** — Exophytic or through renal capsule

Lymphoma — Non-Hodgkin lymphoma

Adrenal mass — Multiplanar evaluation helpful

Urinoma — Collecting system perforation

Pancreatitis — Most frequent source of fluid in anterior pararenal space

*Sarcoma* — Usually from capsule; leiomyosarcoma, liposarcoma, and fibrosarcoma

# GASTROINTESTINAL TRACT

## 122. DILATED ESOPHAGUS

**Normal**

| | |
|---|---|
| **Achalasia** | Absence of Auerbach plexus ganglion cells, increased rate of malignancy |
| **Esophageal carcinoma** | Ulcerating tumor or wall thickening, dilatation proximal to mass |
| Stricture | Following infection, inflammation, caustic ingestion |
| Esophagitis | Thick wall |
| Scleroderma | 80% with esophageal involvement, patulous GEJ, basilar lung disease, dilated small bowel |
| Mediastinitis | Traction |
| Gastric carcinoma | Pseudoachalasia, GEJ mass |
| Diabetic neuropathy | Gastroparesis |

| | |
|---|---|
| Vagotomy | |
| Chagas disease | *Trypanosoma cruzi* infection, neurotoxic to Auerbach plexus |
| *Amyloidosis* | |

# 123. NARROWED ESOPHAGUS

| | |
|---|---|
| **Normal, collapsed** | Can distend with contrast or gas |

## Esophagitis

| | |
|---|---|
| **Reflux** | Most common cause of esophageal strictures, high stricture suggests Barrett esophagus |
| Radiation | Long segment corresponding to therapeutic port |
| Infection/inflammation | *Candida,* tuberculosis, syphilis, Crohn disease very uncommon |
| Drugs | Focal ulcer/stricture; erythromycin, potassium chloride, quinidine |
| Caustic ingestion | Lye or alkali, long segment, increased rate of malignancy |

## Tumors

| | |
|---|---|
| **Esophageal carcinoma** | Infiltrating type may occur over long segment; alcohol, tylosis, and smoking are risk factors |

| | |
|---|---|
| Gastric adenocarcinoma | >90% of gastric malignancies |
| Benign mural masses | Leiomyoma, lipoma, granular cell myoblastoma |
| Invasion by adjacent tumor | Lung cancer |
| Lymphoma | Extension from mediastinal involvement |
| Metastases | |

**Other lesions**

| | |
|---|---|
| Post–nasogastric tube | Long segment, usually distal |
| Diffuse esophageal spasm | Segmental contractions, may cause chest pain |
| Postsurgical | History helpful |
| Schatzki ring | Ring at GEJ, symptoms if <13 mm, usually acquired from reflux |
| Esophageal web | Idiopathic near cricopharyngeus muscle, epidermolysis bullosa, pemphigus, Plummer-Vinson syndrome |

## 124. THICKENED OR NARROWED STOMACH

| | |
|---|---|
| **Incomplete distention** | Can employ contrast, water, or gas crystals |

**Tumors**

| | |
|---|---|
| **Adenocarcinoma** | >90% of gastric malignancies pernicious anemia, achlorhydria, atrophy are risk factors |
| **Lymphoma** | Usually NHL, less rigid than infiltrating gastric cancer |
| Metastases | Infiltrating breast metastases mimic gastric adenocarcinoma; focal from colon, pancreas |

**Inflammation**

| | |
|---|---|
| **Peptic gastritis** | Antral, ulcer history |
| **Pancreatitis** | Posterior wall edema |
| Alcoholic gastritis | May include evidence of fatty liver, cirrhosis, pancreatitis |
| Zollinger-Ellison syndrome | Thick folds, excess fluid, pancreatic gastrinoma |

| | |
|---|---|
| Atrophic gastritis | Diffusely narrowed, decreased folds, pernicious anemia association |
| Infection | *Candida,* CMV, herpes, *Cryptosporidium,* toxoplasmosis |
| Corrosive gastritis | Usually acids, antrum preferentially involved |
| Eosinophilic gastritis | Antral predilection, thick folds 50% with small bowel disease |
| Crohn disease | Uncommon, apthous ulcers |
| *Radiation* | Antral predilection, >5000 rads |
| *Granulomatous disease* | Tuberculosis, syphilis, sarcoid; antral predilection |
| *Menetrier disease* | Spares antrum, small bowel edema from hypoproteinemia |

## Other lesions

| | |
|---|---|
| Lymphoid hyperplasia | Antral |
| Gastric varices | Associated esophageal varices, portal hypertension, or splenic vein thrombosis |
| *Amyloidosis* | |

## 125. GASTRIC MASS

### Malignant tumors

| | |
|---|---|
| **Adenocarcinoma** | >90% of gastric malignancies; pernicious anemia, achlorhydria, atrophy are risk factors |
| **Lymphoma** | Usually NHL, 30% extend into duodenum, less rigid than infiltrating gastric cancer |
| Metastases | Melanoma, lung, breast (infiltrating), Kaposi sarcoma |
| Leiomyosarcoma | Large, ulcerated or necrotic mass; Carney triad of pulmonary chondroma and pheochromocytoma |

### Benign tumors

| | |
|---|---|
| Mesenchymal tumors | Leiomyoma (most common benign tumor), lipoma (fat attenuation) |
| Polyp | Hyperplastic (90%), adenomatous (malignant potential), hamartomatous (Peutz-Jeghers) |

## Other lesions

| | |
|---|---|
| Bezoar | Mobile, vegetable (phytobezoar) or hair (trichobezoar) |
| Surgery | Fundoplication may mimic a mass at GEJ |
| Gastric varices | Serpiginous and enhancing, portal hypertension or splenic vein thrombosis |
| Ectopic pancreatic tissue | Usually greater curve near pylorus, potential central orifice |
| *Hematoma* | Trauma, coagulopathy |

## 126. PNEUMATOSIS INTESTINALIS
(air in bowel wall)

**Idiopathic**

| | |
|---|---|
| **Ischemia/ infarction** | Portal or SMV gas, bowel-wall thickening |
| Ulcerative colitis | Rectum and continuous retrograde involvement, pancolitis in 30%, heterogeneous wall enhancement; increased risk of carcinoma, toxic megacolon, sclerosing cholangitis |
| Recent bowel surgery | |
| Crohn disease | Terminal ileum, fistulae, abscesses, creeping fat |
| Pseudomembranous colitis | Clostridial infection following antibiotic therapy, pancolitis |
| Toxic megacolon | Dilated and thickened bowel; ulcerative colitis, pseudomembranous colitis, *Salmonella,* Crohn disease, ischemia, amebiasis |

| | |
|---|---|
| Graft-vs-host disease | Proximal small bowel, acute or chronic, "ribbon bowel" |
| Perforated diverticulum | Rectosigmoid predilection, abscess, soft tissue infiltration |
| Scleroderma/ dermatomyositis | Wide-mouth diverticula, dilated esophagus, "hidebound small bowel" |
| Necrotizing enterocolitis | Neonates, can be epidemic, may have portal gas and late strictures |
| *COPD* | |

# 127. DILATED SMALL BOWEL

## Obstruction

| | |
|---|---|
| **Adhesions** | 60% of small bowel obstruction, ileum most common; surgery, radiation therapy, prior peritonitis |
| **Hernia** | 95% external |
| Intussusception | Mesenteric fat within lumen, lead mass in adults, celiac disease/scleroderma cause transient intussusceptions |
| Volvulus | Malrotation predisposes |
| Foreign body | Gallstone, ascariasis, foreign body, meconium |
| Stricture | Crohn disease, radiation therapy, ischemia |
| Hematoma | Trauma, coagulopathy, Henoch-Schönlein purpura |

## Ileus

| | |
|---|---|
| **Recent surgery** | First 5 postoperative days |
| **Peritonitis** | Usually associated ascites |

| | |
|---|---|
| **Drugs** | Opiates and sympathomimetic drugs |
| **Intraabdominal inflammation** | Pancreatitis, acute cholecystitis, appendicitis, pyelonephritis |
| Ischemia or vasculitis | Thromboembolic disease, lupus, polyarteritis nodosa |
| Idiopathic pseudo-obstruction | Ogilvie syndrome |
| Electrolyte imbalance | Low potassium or chloride, calcium or magnesium imbalance |
| Gastroenteritis or enterocolitis | Increased intraluminal fluid, wall thickening |
| Shock | "Shock bowel," increased mural enhancement, flattened IVC |
| Celiac disease (nontropical sprue) | Mid- and distal jejunal dilatation, fluid accumulation, contrast dilution |
| Scleroderma | Primarily proximal small bowel, wide-mouth diverticula, transient intussusception |

| | |
|---|---|
| Colonic resection | Compensatory dilatation |
| Amyloidosis | Can produce occult gastrointestinal bleed, obstruction, malabsorption; may precede myeloma |

## 128. THICKENED SMALL BOWEL

### Edema

| | |
|---|---|
| Congestive heart failure | Dilated IVC and hepatic veins, mottled hepatic enhancement |
| Zollinger-Ellison syndrome | Thickened duodenum and proximal small bowel folds, gastrinoma |
| Venous congestion | Thrombosis, mass obstructing venous return (carcinoid) |
| Hypoproteinemia | Nephrotic syndrome, cirrhosis, ascites |
| Lymphatic obstruction | Lymphoma, retroperitoneal fibrosis, surgery |
| *Lymphangectasia* | Ascites, pleural effusions, "halo sign" |
| *Angioneurotic edema* | C1 esterase inhibitor deficiency |

### Inflammation

| | |
|---|---|
| **Pancreatitis** | Adjacent inflammation, sentinel loop of third portion of duodenum |

| | |
|---|---|
| **Crohn disease** | Terminal ileum, fistulae, abscesses, creeping fat |

## Infection/enteritis

| | |
|---|---|
| **Duodenitis** | Peptic ulcer disease, Zollinger-Ellison |
| *Giardia* | Proximal small bowel, hypermotility, increased fluid |
| MAI | Proximal small bowel, low-attenuation adenopathy, HIV patients |
| *Cryptosporidium* | Proximal small bowel, increased fluid, HIV patients |
| Tuberculosis | Ileum and cecum, gastric antrum and pylorus usually involved |
| Strongyloidiasis | Proximal small bowel, "toothpaste bowel" |
| Others | *Yersinia, Candida,* CMV, ascariasis |
| Celiac disease (nontropical sprue) | Generally no thickening; dilatation, fluid accumulation, mesenteric adenopathy |

| | |
|---|---|
| Radiation therapy | Small bowel is very radiosensitive |
| Eosinophilic enteritis | Gastric and proximal small bowel involvement, children and young adults, blood eosinophilia |
| Whipple disease | Low-attenuation adenopathy, thick folds, no dilatation, normal transit time |
| Graft-vs-host disease | Proximal small bowel, acute or chronic, "ribbon bowel" |
| *Behçet* | Focal, mass-like ulcers in the ileum as well as buccal and genital surfaces |

## Tumors

| | |
|---|---|
| **Metastases** | Melanoma, breast, ovary, gastrointestinal, Kaposi sarcoma |
| **Lymphoma** | Associated adenopathy, aneurysmal dilatation, HIV and celiac disease predispose |
| Carcinoid | Most common in appendix (benign) and ileum |

## Other lesions

| | |
|---|---|
| **Ischemia** | Vasculitis, thromboembolism; postprandial pain is a common symptom in chronic cases |
| **Hemorrhage** | Trauma, coagulopathy, Henoch-Schönlein purpura |
| *Mastocytosis* | Sclerotic bones, reticuloendothelial system involvement |
| *Amyloidosis* | Diffuse or focal, decreased motility, adenopathy or other organ involvement, no dilatation |

# 129. THICKENED TERMINAL ILEUM

## Inflammation

| | |
|---|---|
| **Crohn disease** | 80% have ileal involvement, 30% with small bowel disease only, creeping fat, abscesses, fistulae |
| **Appendicitis** | Soft tissue stranding, abscess, 25% with appendicolith |
| Ulcerative colitis | Backwash ileitis, 10% of patients |
| Radiation therapy | Small bowel is very radiosensitive |

## Infection

| | |
|---|---|
| **Yersinia** | Associated ascending colon involvement, mimics appendicitis |
| *Salmonella* | Associated ascending colon involvement, diarrhea |
| Tuberculosis | Associated cecal involvement, CXR generally normal |
| CMV | Ulcers and fistulae, HIV patients |

## Tumors

| | |
|---|---|
| Lymphoma | Most common small bowel malignancy, distal small bowel, 80% solitary, celiac disease association |
| Carcinoid | Distal ileum/appendix, may be multiple, desmoplastic nodes with tethering |

## Other lesions

| | |
|---|---|
| Ischemia/infarction | Acute presentation, thromboembolic disease |
| *Hematoma* | Trauma, anticoagulation, ITP, hemophilia |

# 130. SMALL BOWEL MASS

## Malignant tumors

| | |
|---|---|
| **Lymphoma** | Most common small bowel malignancy, distal small bowel, 80% solitary, celiac disease association |
| **Adenocarcinoma** | Proximal small bowel; celiac disease, Peutz-Jeghers, Crohn disease association |
| **Metastases** | Melanoma, breast, lung, Kaposi sarcoma |
| Leiomyosarcoma | Ileum most common, large mass, may have ulceration |

## Benign tumors

| | |
|---|---|
| **Leiomyoma** | Most common benign small bowel tumor |
| **Lipoma** | Ileum, fat attenuation |
| **Carcinoid** | Distal ileum/appendix, may be multiple, desmoplastic response with tethering |

| | |
|---|---|
| Hemangioma | Jejunum and ileum; multiple and sessile; tuberous sclerosis, Osler-Weber-Rendu |
| Adenoma | 60% tubular, 40% villous |
| Polyps | Adenomatous, hamartomatous, inflammatory<br>Peutz-Jeghers—hamartomatous, no malignant potential<br>Gardner—small bowel and colon adenomatous polyps, ampullary tumor, invariable colon malignancy<br>Cronkhite-Canada—inflammatory, fold thickening and increased small bowel fluid |

## Other lesions

| | |
|---|---|
| Duplication cyst | Proximal small bowel, water attenuation |
| Hematoma | Variable density depending on age |

## 131. ENLARGED, DISTENDED COLON

| | |
|---|---|
| **Mechanical obstruction** | Cancer, intussusception, diverticulitis |
| **Ileus** | Sepsis, electrolyte imbalance, surgery, peritonitis, appendicitis, pancreatitis, shock |
| Drugs | Chemotherapy, NSAIDs, antihypertensives |
| Functional | Idiopathic pseudoobstruction |
| Infarction | Associated bowel-wall thickening |
| Electrolyte imbalance | Low potassium, chloride, calcium |
| Toxic megacolon | Dilated and thickened; ulcerative colitis, pseudomembranous colitis, *Salmonella,* Crohn disease, ischemia, amebiasis |
| Scleroderma | Wide-mouth diverticula, dilated esophagus, "hidebound small bowel" |
| Laxative abuse | Ahaustral descending colon |

## 132. COLONIC OBSTRUCTION

| | |
|---|---|
| **Intussusception** | Lead mass in adults, doughnut sign with central fat |
| **Diverticulitis** | Rectum and continuous retrograde involvement, pancolitis in 30%; rule out underlying cancer |
| **Colon cancer** | Usually focal, CT is sensitive in detecting adjacent adenopathy, invasion beyond wall |
| **Fecal impaction** | Elderly or paralyzed patients |
| Ulcerative colitis | Rectum and continuous retrograde involvement; increased risk of carcinoma, toxic megacolon, sclerosing cholangitis |
| Crohn disease | Usually with ileal involvement as well; creeping fat, abscesses, skip lesions |
| Adhesions | Prior surgery, bowel tethering |

## 133. THICKENED COLON

### Inflammation

**Diverticulitis** — Soft tissue stranding, abscess, perforation, sigmoid predilection, rule out underlying cancer

**Ulcerative colitis** — Rectum and continuous retrograde involvement, pancolitis in 30%, heterogeneous wall enhancement; increased risk of carcinoma, toxic megacolon, sclerosing cholangitis

**Pseudomembranous colitis** — Clostridial infection following antibiotic therapy, pancolitis

Crohn disease — 50% of Crohn patients with small bowel and colonic disease; creeping fat, abscesses

Typhlitis — Immunocompromised patients, cecum and ascending colon

| | |
|---|---|
| Infectious colitis | Left colon—*Shigella*, schistosomiasis; right colon—*Salmonella*, tuberculosis, *Yersinia*, amebiasis; pancolitis—CMV, *Campylobacter* |
| Toxic megacolon | 10% of ulcerative colitis patients; also Crohn disease, CMV, ischemia, pseudomembranous colitis, amebiasis |

## Tumor

| | |
|---|---|
| **Adenocarcinoma** | Usually focal, CT has low sensitivity in detecting adjacent adenopathy, invasion beyond wall |
| Lymphoma | Primary NHL in HIV, can infiltrate long segment or be more focal |
| Metastases | Melanoma, breast, lung, Kaposi sarcoma |

## Other lesions

| | |
|---|---|
| Hematoma | Trauma, anticoagulation |

| | |
|---|---|
| Ischemic colitis | Follows vascular distribution: IMA>SMA>watershed |
| Radiation | Generally rectosigmoid, ulcers and fistulae |
| Amyloidosis | Can produce occult gastrointestinal bleed, obstruction, small bowel malabsorption; may precede multiple myeloma |
| *Angioneurotic edema* | C1 esterase inhibitor deficiency |

## 134. COLONIC MASS

### Polyps

| | |
|---|---|
| **Hypertrophic** | Most common, no malignant potential |
| **Adenomatous** | Tubular, tubulovillous, and villous types; malignant progression; familial, Gardner, Turcot |
| Hamartomatous | No malignant potential; Peutz-Jeghers, Gardner, Cowden, Cronkhite-Canada |
| Juvenile | Juvenile polyposis |

### Tumors

| | |
|---|---|
| **Adenocarcinoma** | Usually focal, CT has low sensitivity in detecting adjacent adenopathy, invasion beyond wall |
| Lymphoma | Primary NHL in HIV, can infiltrate long segment or be more focal |
| Metastases | Melanoma, breast, lung, Kaposi sarcoma |

| | |
|---|---|
| Carcinoid | 90% of appendiceal tumors, desmoplastic mesenteric nodes, syndrome implies hepatic metastases |
| Stromal tumors | Leiomyoma, lipoma, hemangioma |
| Mucocele | Can progress to mucinous cystadenoma/carcinoma, can yield pseudomyxoma peritonei |

**Other lesions**

| | |
|---|---|
| Hematoma | Trauma, coagulopathy |

# 135. NARROWED CECUM

## Inflammation

**Crohn disease** — 80% of Crohn patients have small bowel involvement, 50% with small bowel and colonic disease; creeping fat, abscesses

**Appendicitis** — Soft tissue stranding, abscess, 25% with appendicolith

Ulcerative colitis — Rectum and continuous retrograde involvement, pancolitis in 30%

Typhlitis — Immunocompromised patients

## Infection

*Yersinia* — Associated ascending colon involvement, mimics appendicitis

*Salmonella* — Associated ascending colon involvement, diarrhea

Tuberculosis — Associated ascending colon/ileal involvement, low-

|   |   |
|---|---|
|   | attenuation adenopathy, CXR generally normal |
| Amebiasis | Associated ascending colon involvement, skip lesions, rare ameboma |

**Tumors**

|   |   |
|---|---|
| **Adenocarcinoma** | Usually focal, CT has low sensitivity in detecting adjacent adenopathy, invasion beyond wall |
| Carcinoid | 90% of appendiceal tumors, desmoplastic mesenteric nodes, syndrome implies hepatic metastases |
| Mucocele | Can progress to mucinous cystadenoma/carcinoma, can yield pseudomyxoma peritonei |
| Metastases | Melanoma, breast, lung, Kaposi sarcoma |

# GENITOURINARY TRACT

## 136. URETRAL DILATATION

| | |
|---|---|
| **Obstruction** | Stone, tumor/adjacent mass, inflammation, blood clot, fungus ball, ectopic ureterocele |
| **Vesicoureteral reflux** | Pediatric patients, urinary diversions |
| Primary megaloureter | Absent distal ureteral peristalsis |
| *Prune belly syndrome* | Congenital nonhereditary, usually male |

## 137. DIFFUSE BLADDER-WALL THICKENING

| | |
|---|---|
| **Nondistended bladder** | >300 mL for adequate CT cystogram |
| **Outlet obstruction** | Prostatic enlargement most commonly |

### Cystitis

| | |
|---|---|
| **Radiation** | Acute changes resolve in 12 to 18 months |
| Infection | Tuberculosis, viral, fungal |
| Inflammatory | Cystitis cystica and glandularis (premalignant) |

### Other

| | |
|---|---|
| Adjacent inflammation | Diverticulitis, PID |
| Neurogenic bladder | Dilation, sacculation |

# 138. BLADDER CALCIFICATION

| | |
|---|---|
| **Calculus** | Stasis, outlet obstruction |
| Drug-induced cystitis | Cyclophosphamide |
| Prior radiation therapy | Acute changes resolve in 12 to 18 months, calcification usually later |
| Schistosomiasis | Most common cause worldwide, hematogenous spread to distal ureters/bladder |
| Foreign body | Foley balloon fragment |
| *Adenocarcinoma* | Urachal cancer at anterosuperior bladder with mucous micturition in 25%, bladder extrophy |
| *Transitional cell carcinoma* | Smoking, aniline dyes, cyclophosphamide predispose |
| *Squamous cell carcinoma* | Schistosomiasis infection, stricture, calculi predipose |
| *Tuberculosis* | Upper genitourinary tract invariably involved |

## 139. FILLING DEFECT IN BLADDER

| | |
|---|---|
| **Foreign body** | Particularly Foley catheter |
| **Blood clot** | Evaluate for trauma, tumor, stone, intervention |
| **Enlarged prostate** | Median lobe hypertrophy with BPH, prostate contiguity |
| Calculus | Stasis, outlet obstruction |
| Primary tumor | Transitional cell, 5% squamous cell, 2% adenocarcinoma; embryonal rhabdomyosarcoma in children; rare pheochromocytoma at base |
| Ureterocele | Duplication, "cobra head" |
| Fungus ball | Diabetic predisposition |

## 140. AIR IN BLADDER WALL OR LUMEN

| | |
|---|---|
| **Instrumentation** | Catheterization, cystoscopy, ureteroscopy |
| **Trauma** | CT cystogram with >300 mL to exclude bladder rupture |
| **Fistula** | Colon, small bowel, vagina; radiation, cancer, Crohn disease, diverticulitis, surgery predispose |
| Emphysematous cystitis | *E. coli* infection in diabetics |

## 141. CALCIFIED SEMINAL VESICLES AND VAS DEFERENS

**Diabetes mellitus** Most common cause

**Idiopathic**

Chronic infection or inflammation — Tuberculosis—upper gastrointestinal tract invariably involved; schistosomiasis—hematogenous spread

## 142. PELVIC FLUID (CUL-DE-SAC)

| | |
|---|---|
| **Normal** | <50 mL |
| **Ovulation** | May have mittelschmertz, correlate with menstrual cycle |
| Ectopic pregnancy | Possible high attenuation of acute hemorrhage, adnexal mass |
| Ovarian neoplasm | Adnexal mass, cystic or solid |
| Pelvic inflammatory disease | Hydrosalpinx, tuboovarian abscess |
| Peritonitis | Ascites, enhancing peritoneum |
| Cirrhosis | Nodular liver, small right lobe, findings of portal hypertension |
| Appendicitis | Soft tissue stranding, abscess, 25% with appendicolith |
| Ascites from other causes | Differential 74 |

## 143. ENLARGED UTERUS

| | |
|---|---|
| **Leiomyomata (fibroids)** | Most common uterine mass, 25% of women, multiple and often calcify |
| **Adenomyosis** | Focal or diffuse endometrial invasion of myometrium, can cause dysmenorrhea, association with endometriosis |
| **Obstruction** | Low-density center postcontrast; cervical stenosis, cervical carcinoma, polyps |
| **Endometrial carcinoma** | >90% adenocarcinoma, direct invasion and pelvic nodal spread |
| Pyometra | Usually obstructing lesion, associated with squamous cell endometrial cancer |
| Endometrial hyperplasia | Postmenopausal women with unopposed estrogen, two forms with adenomatous type premalignant |
| Endometrial polyps | 20% multiple, <4% malignant transformation |

| | |
|---|---|
| Hydatidiform mole | Spectrum with choriocarcinoma as malignant form, elevated $\beta$-HCG |
| Pregnancy | Intrauterine fetus |
| *Leiomyosarcoma* | Heterogeneous invasive mass |

## 144. SOLID OVARIAN MASS

| | |
|---|---|
| **Epithelial tumors** | 95% of ovarian malignancies; nulliparity, family history, age predispose |
| **Serous cystadenoma carcinoma** | 30% of ovarian tumors, 40% malignant; large, cystic masses with ascites |
| **Mucinous cystadenoma carcinoma** | 20% of ovarian tumors, 20% malignant; large, cystic masses with ascites, may lead to pseudomyxoma peritonei |
| Endometroid carcinoma | 20% of ovarian malignancies |
| Rare epithelial tumors | Clear cell; Brenner; cystadenofibroma |
| **Germ cell tumors** | 1 to 2% of ovarian malignancies |
| **Dermoid** | Most common benign ovarian tumor; variable fat, cystic, solid, and calcific components; 10 to 15% bilateral |

| | |
|---|---|
| Dysgerminoma | 75% <30 years old, 2% of ovarian malignancies, radiosensitive |
| Endodermal sinus tumor | Children and young women, poor prognosis |
| Immature teratoma | Malignant, late detection and poor prognosis |
| **Stromal tumors** | 2 to 3% of ovarian malignancies |
| Granulosa or thecal cell tumor | 5% of ovarian tumors; precocious puberty in children, endometrial carcinoma and cystic breast disease in adults |
| Fibroma | Meig syndrome with ascites and right-sided pleural effusion, basal cell nevus syndrome |
| Choriocarcinoma | Malignant gestational trophoblastic disease; hypervascular with hematogenous metastases to lung, kidneys, and brain |
| Sertoli-Leydig cell tumor | Masculinizing tumor |

## Other lesions

| | |
|---|---|
| Endometrioma | Complex, potentially high-attenuation fluid, which may have fluid-fluid levels |
| Metastases | 5% of ovarian masses; breast, bowel, endometrial, skin primaries; mucin-containing Krukenberg tumors |
| Ovarian torsion | More common in young women, often with cyst/tumor, free fluid |
| Oophoritis | Enlarged, low attenuation |
| Nongynecologic | Hematoma, abscess |
| *Sarcoma* | Fibrosarcoma |

## 145. CYSTIC OVARIAN MASS

| | |
|---|---|
| **Physiologic cysts** | May be hemorrhagic; follicular cyst—>2.5 cm, follow up in 6 to 8 weeks with ultrasound, no follow up needed if <2.5 cm and premenopausal; corpus luteum cyst—larger, symptomatic; theca lutein cyst—large, usually bilateral, 50% associated with trophoblastic disease |
| **Tuboovarian abscess/PID** | Tubular with thick, enhancing wall, adjacent inflammatory change |
| **Cystadenoma or cystadenocarcinoma** | 30% of ovarian tumors, 40% malignant; large, cystic masses with ascites; nulliparity, family history, age predispose |
| Dermoid | Most common benign ovarian tumor; variable fat, cystic, solid, and calcific components; 25% bilateral, |

| | |
|---|---|
| | dermoid plug (Rokitansky mural nodule in cystic dermoid) |
| Ectopic pregnancy | Often with high-attenuation free fluid, check $\beta$-HCG |
| Hydrosalpinx | Tubular |
| Endometrioma | Complex cystic mass, may seed laparoscopy site |
| Paraadnexal lesion | Lymphocele |
| Hyperstimulated ovary | Multiple, small peripheral cysts |
| *Epithelial inclusion cyst* | |

## 146. CALCIFIED OVARIAN LESION

**Dermoid**
Most common benign ovarian tumor; variable fat, cystic, solid, and calcific components; 10 to 15% bilateral

**Cystadenoma/ cystadeno- carcinoma**
30% of ovarian tumors, 40% malignant; large, cystic masses with ascites; nulliparity, family history, age predispose

*Hemangioperi- cytoma*

# CHEST AND ABDOMINAL WALL

## 147. GYNECOMASTIA

| | |
|---|---|
| **Drugs** | Estrogen, digitalis, marijuana, tricyclic antidepressants, reserpine, thiazides |
| **Cirrhosis** | Small, irregular liver, ascites |
| Chronic renal failure with hemodialysis | |
| Senile | Decreased serum testosterone |
| Tumor | Adrenal, testicular, or pituitary tumors with hormonal activity |
| Adrenal | Lesions affecting adrenal cortex |
| Chronic lung disease | Especially emphysema |
| Hypogonadism or hypopituitarism | Decreased serum testosterone |

## 148. BODY-WALL MASS

**Sebaceous cyst** In subcutaneous tissue

**Hematoma** Decreases in size and attenuation over time, can calcify

### Tumors

Bone — Multiple myeloma, metastases, chondrosarcoma, Ewing sarcoma, others

Soft tissue — Lymphoma, melanoma, bronchogenic carcinoma; sarcomas including MFH, fibrosarcoma, rhabdosarcoma, liposarcoma, or neurofibrosarcoma

Benign tumor — Lipoma, fibroma, hibernoma, hemangioma—phleboliths and tortuous vessels, elastofibroma, desmoid, neurofibroma, schwannoma, dermoid, exostosis

## Infection

| | |
|---|---|
| Bacteria | *Actinomyces, Nocardia, Staphylococcus* |
| Fungus | Blastomycosis, aspergillosis |
| Tuberculosis | Uncommon, may calcify |

# 149. SOFT TISSUE CALCIFICATIONS

| | |
|---|---|
| **Scleroderma** | Basilar lung disease, esophageal dysmotility, "wide-mouthed diverticulae" of bowel |
| **Trauma** | Myositis ossificans, thermal and electrical injuries, fat necrosis |
| **Injection granulomata** | Usually gluteal |
| **Vascular disease** | Atherosclerosis, venous phleboliths |
| Hypercalcemia | Hyperparathyroidism, renal osteodystrophy, widespread osseous metastases, excess vitamin D, immobilization, sarcoid |
| Metabolic disease | Hypo/pseudo/pseudopseudo-hypoparathyroidism, CPPD, gout, diabetes |
| CREST syndrome | Calcinosis, Raynaud, esophageal dysmotility, sclerodactyly, telangectasia |

| | |
|---|---|
| Dermatomyositis | Sheet-like calcification and muscular atrophy, also other collagen vascular diseases |
| Hemangioma | Small round calcifications—phleboliths |
| Calcified lymph nodes | |
| Calcinosis | May be joint-centered "tumoral calcinosis" |
| Degenerating fibroadenoma | Breast lesion |
| Chondrosarcoma | From osteochondromas, chondral junctions such as anterior ribs |
| *Parasites* | Cysticercosis, other worms |
| *Osteosarcoma* | Rarely extraosseous |

## 150. SCLEROTIC BONE LESION

**Bone island** — Enostosis; dense, focal, well marginated; ileum most common

**Metastasis** — Often breast or prostate cancer, lymphoma; treated lytic lesion

**Healing fracture** — New bone formation and periosteal reaction

Osteochondroma — Exostosis, benign but potential malignant transformation with pain or cartilage cap >2 cm (up to 3 cm in child)

Osteonecrosis/infarct — Idiopathic, steroids, alcohol, sickle cell, vasculitis, trauma, Caisson disease

Benign lesion — Osteoma, healing nonossifying fibroma, ossifying fibroma, enchondroma, osteoid osteoma

Infection — Chronic osteomyelitis, sclerosing osteomyelitis of Garré

| | |
|---|---|
| Primary malignancy | Osteosarcoma, Ewing sarcoma (especially flat bones) |
| Fibrous dysplasia | Medullary bone replaced with "woven" bone; ribs, proximal femur; most <30 years old; polyostotic form may have café-au-lait spots and endocrine abnormalities (McCune-Albright) |
| Paget disease | Bone enlargement, thickened trabeculae, often mixed sclerosis and lysis; often polyostotic with pelvis, spine, and proximal femur most common |

## 151. LYTIC BONE LESION

### Malignancy

| | |
|---|---|
| **Hematogenous metastasis** | Renal cell, thyroid cancer, lung cancer, lymphoma, neuroblastoma |
| **Multiple myeloma** or plasmacytoma | Spine, pelvis, skull, and ribs; associated anemia, diffuse osteopenia, renal failure, and amyloid |
| Direct extension | Lung cancer, sarcomas, others |
| Primary bone tumor | Ewing sarcoma, chondrosarcoma, fibrosarcoma, lymphoma |

### Other

| | |
|---|---|
| Osteomyelitis | *Staphylococcus,* tuberculosis, actinomycosis, *Nocardia;* may form Brodie abscess, sequestrum |
| Benign tumor | Nonossifying fibroma, enchondroma, Langerhans cell histiocytosis, giant cell tumor, osteoblastoma, brown |

| | |
|---|---|
| | tumor, chondroblastoma, chondromyxoid fibroma, intraosseous lipoma |
| Fibrous dysplasia | Medullary bone replaced with "woven" bone; ribs, proximal femur; most <30 years old; polyostotic form may have café-au-lait spots and endocrine abnormalities (McCune-Albright) |
| Paget disease | Bone enlargement, thickened trabeculae, often mixed sclerosis and lysis; often polyostotic with pelvis, spine, and femur most common |
| Cysts | Subchondral geodes, aneurysmal bone cyst, unicameral bone cyst |
| Fracture | Linear, potentially with resorption at fracture site |

## 152. DIFFUSE SCLEROSIS

| | |
|---|---|
| **Widespread metastases** | Generally breast or prostate |
| **Sickle cell disease** | Calcified spleen, gallstones, bone infarcts, cardiomegaly |
| **Renal osteodystrophy** | Small kidneys, "rugger jersey spine," potential acquired cystic disease if on dialysis |
| Mastocytosis | Thick trabeculae, often areas of rarefaction; hepatomegaly, adenopathy |
| Myelofibrosis | Anemia, weakness, weight loss; associated splenomegaly, extramedullary hematopoiesis |
| Melorheostosis | Sclerosis along cortex in scleratomal distribution, often painful; also osteopathia striata and osteopoikilosis |
| Paget disease | Bone enlargement, thickened trabeculae, often mixed sclerosis and lysis; often polyostotic with pelvis, spine, and femur most common |

| | |
|---|---|
| Neurocutaneous syndromes | Neurofibromatosis, tuberous sclerosis; associated hyperostosis |
| Osteopetrosis | Inherited dysfunction; dense bones, "sandwich vertebrae," Erlenmeyer-flask deformity; complicated by fractures, anemia |
| *Fluorosis* | More commonly ligamentous calcification |
| *Pyknodysostosis* | Autosomal recessive dwarfism, thick skull base, penciled digits, hypoplastic sinuses |

# BIBLIOGRAPHY

# BIBLIOGRAPHY

Armstrong P, Wilson AG, Dee P, Hansell DM. *Imaging of Diseases of the Chest.* 2nd ed. St. Louis: Mosby–Year Book; 1995.

Burgener FA, Kormano M. *Differential Diagnosis in Conventional Radiology.* New York: Thieme Medical Publishers; 1991.

Burgener FA, Kormano M. *Differential Diagnosis in Computed Tomography.* New York: Thieme Medical Publishers; 1996.

Chapman S, Nakielny R. *Aids to Radiological Differential Diagnosis.* 3rd ed. Philadelphia: WB Saunders; 1995.

Cotran RS, Kumar V, Robbins SL, Schoen FJ. *Robbins Pathologic Basis of Disease.* 5th ed. Philadelphia: WB Saunders; 1994.

Eisenberg RL. *Clinical Imaging: An Atlas of Differential Diagnosis.* 3rd ed. Philadelphia: Lippincott-Raven; 1997.

Fraser RS, Paré JAP, Fraser RG, Paré PD. *Synopsis of Diseases of the Chest.* 2nd ed. Philadelphia: WB Saunders; 1994.

Grainger RG, Allison DJ. *Diagnostic Radiology—A Textbook of Medical Imaging.* 3rd ed. New York: Churchill Livingstone, 1997. Vols 1–3.

Haaga JR, Lanzieri CF, Sartoris DJ, Zerhouni EA. *Computed Tomography and Magnetic Resonance Imaging of the Whole Body.* 3rd ed. St Louis: Mosby–Year Book; 1994. Vols 1–2.

Lee JKT, Sagel SS, Stanley RJ, Heiken JP. *Computed Body Tomography with MRI Correlation.* 3rd ed. Philadelphia: Lippincott-Raven; 1998.

Moss AA, Gamsu G, Genant HK. *Computed Tomography of the Body with Magnetic Resonance Imaging.* 2nd ed. Philadelphia: WB Saunders; 1992. Vols 1–3.

Reed JC. *Chest Radiology—Plain Film Patterns and Differential Diagnosis.* 4th ed. St. Louis: Mosby; 1997.

Reeders JWAJ, Mathieson JR. *AIDS Imaging—A Practical Clinical Approach.* Philadelphia: WB Saunders; 1998.

Silverman FN, Kuhn JP. *Essentials of Caffey's Pediatric X-ray Diagnosis.* Chicago: Year Book Medical Publishers; 1990.

Slone RM, Gutierrez FR, Fisher AJ. *Thoracic Imaging: A Practical Approach.* McGraw-Hill; 1999.

Sutton D. *Textbook of Radiology and Imaging.* 6th ed. New York: Churchill Livingstone; 1998. Vols 1–2.

Webb WR, Müller NL, Naidich DP. *High-Resolution CT of the Lung.* 2nd ed. Philadelphia: Lippincott-Raven; 1996.

Weissleder R, Rieumont MJ, Wittenberg J. *Primer of Diagnostic Imaging.* 2nd ed. St. Louis: Mosby; 1997.

# INDEX

# A

Abdominal abscess, 187–189
Abdominal wall. *See* Chest and abdominal wall
Abscess
  abdominal, 187–189
  lung, 60, 65
  neck mass, 12, 15
  tuboovarian, 324
Accidents. *See* Trauma
Achalasia, 280
Active granulomatous disease, 43
Adenocarcinoma, 246, 284, 286, 299, 304, 306, 309
Adenoid cystic carcinoma, 27
Adenoma, 18, 252
Adenomyomatosis, 229
Adenomyosis, 319
Adenopathy
  calcified lymph nodes, 5–6
  diffuse interstitial disease with, 96–97
  hilar enlargement and, 151–154
  hypervascular lymph nodes, 9
  low-attenuation adenopathy, 7–8
  lymph node dimensions (reference table), 4
  neck mass, 13, 15
  pulmonary nodules with, 85
  retroperitoneal mass, 194
Adhesions, 290
Adrenal glands
  calcification, 254–255
  mass, 252–253
    benign tumors, 252
    malignant tumors, 252–253
Adult polycystic kidney disease (APCKD), 217, 245, 274
Aging
  dilated common bile duct without obstruction, 225
  pancreatic fatty change, 242
Air in bladder wall or lumen, 316
Airspace disease
  chronic lobar consolidation, 104–106
  diffuse pulmonary consolidation, 107–109
  focal or multifocal consolidation, 98–101
  nodular pattern, 102–103
  pulmonary hemorrhage, 110–111
Airway inflammation, 124–125
Alcohol, fatty liver and, 204
Angiomyolipoma, 270, 273
Anterior mediastinal mass, 157–159

Aortic aneurysm, 160, 167, 179
Aortic stenosis, 179
Aortic valve calcifications, 177
APCKD (adult polycystic kidney disease), 217, 245, 274
Appendicitis, 187, 297, 308
ARDS, 92, 107–108
Arteriosclerosis, 259
Asbestos exposure, 142–143
Ascending aortic aneurysm, 160
Ascites, 185–186, 189, 228
Aspiration, 98
  repeated, 105–106
Asymmetric lung size, 50
Atelectasis, 45
  pulmonary collapse and, 51
Atherosclerotic disease, 265
Atherosclerotic splenic artery, 240
Atrial septal defect, 174

## B

Bacterial infection, 33, 98, 113
Barotrauma, 128, 150
Bertin, column of, 271
Bilateral large kidneys, 262–264
Bilateral small kidneys, 259
Bile ducts. *See* Gallbladder and bile ducts
Bladder
  air in bladder wall or lumen, 316
  calcification, 314
  diffuse bladder-wall thickening, 313
  filling defect in, 315
Bland thrombus, 175
Blebs, 69
Blood clot (bladder), 315
Boardmanship, Fleishman's 10 rules of, 1–2
Body-wall mass, 329–330
Bone island, 333
Bronchial narrowing or obstruction, 105
Bronchiectasis, 52–53, 69, 105, 110
Bronchiolitis, 125
Bronchitis, 110
Bronchoalveolar cell carcinoma, 104
Bronchogenic cancer, 59
Bronchogenic carcinoma, 27, 55, 63, 66, 151, 161, 182
Bronchopneumonia, 107, 119
Bullae, 48, 69

## C

Calcification
  adrenal glands, 254–255

Calcification (*Continued*):
  bladder, 314
  cardiac, 177–178
  chest and abdominal wall, soft tissue, 331–332
  hepatic, 206–207
  lymph nodes, 5–6
  ovarian lesion, 326
  pancreas, 243–244
  pleural, 143
  pulmonary nodules, 86–87
  renal, 265–267
  seminal vesicles and vas deferens, 317
  spleen, 240
  vascular, 243
Calculus, 314
Carcinoid, 299
Carcinoma
  bronchogenic, 27, 55, 63, 66, 151, 161, 182
  endometrial, 319
  esophageal, 280, 282
  hepatocellular, 198, 208, 219
  ovarian, 321
  renal, 269, 277
Carcinomatosis, 185
Cardiac and vascular diagnoses
  cardiac calcifications, 177–178
  cardiac mass, 175
  cardiomegaly, 172–174
  pleural effusion with, 140–141
  enlarged ascending aorta, 179
  enlarged pulmonary arteries, 180–181
  enlarged superior vena cava, 182
  pericardial effusion, 176
Cardiophrenic angle mass, 155–156
  abdominal, 156
  mediastinal, 155–156
  pleural, 156
  pulmonary, 156
Cavitary lung lesion, 65–68
  congenital, 66–67
  inflammatory, 65
  tumor, 66
  vascular, 67–68
Cavitary nodules, multiple, 79–81
CBD stone, 226, 229
Cecum, narrowed, 308–309
Chest and abdominal wall
  body-wall mass, 329–330
  diffuse sclerosis, 337–338
  gynecomastia, 328
  lytic bone lesion, 335–336
  sclerotic bone lesion, 333–334
  soft tissue calcifications, 331–332
  trauma, 133, 331
Cholecystitis, 228

Cholelithiasis, 224, 230
Chronic lobar consolidation, 104–106
  recurrent pneumonia, 105–106
Chylothorax, 133–134
Cirrhosis, 185, 200, 328
Coal worker's pneumoconiosis, 83
Colon
  cancer, 302
  enlarged, distended, 301
  mass, 306–307
  obstruction, 302
  thickened, 303–305
Column of Bertin, 271
Compensatory hyperinflation, 48
Congenital hypoplasia, kidney, 258
Congestive heart failure, 30, 131, 135, 138, 140, 172, 182, 185
Consolidation
  chronic lobar, 104–106
  diffuse pulmonary, 107–109
Coronary arteries, 177
Cor pulmonale, 173
Cortical cysts, 274
Crohn disease, 187, 294, 297, 308
Cystadenocarcinoma, 324, 326
Cystadenoma, 324, 326

Cystic fibrosis, 26, 38, 129, 242
Cysts
  liver, 208, 211–212, 215, 217–218
  neck, 15–16
  ovaries, 324–325
  pulmonary. *See* Lung, pulmonary cysts and nodules
  renal, 274–276
  spleen, 237, 239

# D

Dermoid tumors, 321, 326
Diabetes mellitus, 262, 317
Diffuse bladder-wall thickening, 313
Diffuse gallbladder-wall thickening, 228
Diffuse interstitial lung disease, 88–90
  acute, 88
  with adenopathy, 96–97
  chronic, 88–90
  with pleural effusion, 95
Diffuse lung disease, 30–37
  interstitial. *See* Diffuse interstitial lung disease
  with normal or increased lung volumes, 38
  opportunistic infections, 33–34

Diffuse lung disease (*Continued*):
  pneumonia, 31–32
  pneumothorax and, 129–130
  pulmonary edema, 30–31
  tumor, 34
Diffuse pulmonary consolidation, 107–109
Diffuse sclerosis, 337–338
Dilated common bile duct without obstruction, 225
Dilated esophagus, 280–281
Dilated small bowel, 290–292
  ileus, 290–291
  obstruction, 290
Distended colon, 301
Diverticulitis, 187, 302–303
Dromedary hump, 271
Duodenitis, 294
Duplication cyst, 163, 168

## E

Emphysema, 38, 48
Empyema, 143
Endobronchial mass, 27
Enlarged ascending aorta, 179
Enlarged colon, 301
Enlarged gallbladder, 224
Enlarged parotid gland, 20–21
Enlarged prostate, 315
Enlarged pulmonary arteries, 180–181
Enlarged right atrium, 155
Enlarged superior vena cava, 182
  obstruction, 182
Enlarged uterus, 319–320
Epithelial tumors (ovaries), 321
Esophagitis, 282
Esophagus
  dilated, 166, 280–281
  narrowed, 282–283
Eventration of hemidiaphragm, 50
Extrapleural fat deposition, 142
Extrapleural lesion, 148
Exudate, 132

## F

Fasting, 224
Fat
  liver, 198, 202, 204, 208, 212, 216, 220
  mediastinum, 157, 168
  pancreatic fatty change, 242
  pericardial, 155
Fecal impaction, 302
Fibrosing alveolitis, 112
Fibrosis, 43, 52, 88
  with honeycombing, 69–70
  retroperitoneum, 193

Filling defect in bladder, 315
Fistula, 316
Fleishman's 10 rules of boardmanship, 1–2
Fluid collection, 168
Fluid overload, 30, 131, 138
Focal gallbladder-wall thickening, 229
Focal lung disease
  pneumothorax and, 128–129
Focal nodular hyperplasia, 221
Focal or multifocal
  consolidation, 98–101
  infection, 98–99
Foreign body (bladder), 315

## G

Gallbladder and bile ducts
  diffuse gallbladder-wall thickening, 228
  dilated common bile duct without obstruction, 225
  enlarged gallbladder, 224
  focal gallbladder-wall thickening, 229
  gallbladder carcinoma, 229
  high-attenuation bile, 230
  intrahepatic biliary dilatation, 226–227
  pneumobilia, 231
Gallstone passage, 231
Gastric mass, 286–287
Gastrointestinal tract
  colonic mass, 306–307
  colonic obstruction, 302
  dilated esophagus, 280–281
  dilated small bowel, 290–292
  enlarged, distended colon, 301
  gastric mass, 286–287
  narrowed cecum, 308–309
  narrowed esophagus, 282–283
  pneumatosis intestinalis, 288–289
  small bowel mass, 299–300
  thickened colon, 303–305
  thickened or narrowed stomach, 284–285
  thickened small bowel, 293–296
  thickened terminal ileum, 297–298
Genitourinary tract
  air in bladder wall or lumen, 316
  bladder calcification, 314
  calcified ovarian lesion, 326
  calcified seminal vesicles and vas deferens, 317
  cystic ovarian mass, 324–325
  diffuse bladder-wall thickening, 313

Genitourinary tract (*Continued*):
  enlarged uterus, 319–320
  filling defect in bladder, 315
  pelvic fluid (cul-de-sac), 318
  solid ovarian mass, 321–323
  ureteral dilatation, 312
Germ cell tumors, 157, 321–322
Global pulmonary patterns. *See* Lung, global pulmonary patterns
Glomerulonephritis, 259, 266
Goiter, 18
Gram negative bacteria, 32
Gram positive bacteria, 31–32
Granulomatous disease, 5, 54, 63, 76, 82, 85–86, 102, 119, 151, 154, 206, 240
Ground-glass opacities, 112–114
  infection, 113–114
Gynecomastia, 328

# H

Hamartoma, 56, 59, 61
Healing fracture, 333
Hemangioma, 209, 211, 213, 219, 237
Hematoma, 148, 194, 238, 277, 329
Hemidiaphragm, eventration of, 50
Hemolytic anemia, 235
Hemorrhage
  adrenal glands, 254
  peritoneum, 193
  pulmonary, 108, 110–111
  small bowel, 296
Hemothorax, 133, 143
Hepatic calcifications, 206–207
Hepatic congestion, 199, 202
Hepatocellular carcinoma, 198, 208, 219
Hepatomegaly, 198–201
  hepatic congestion, 199
  primary tumor, 198–199
Hernia, 290
High-attenuation bile, 230
High-output heart disease, 172
Hila. *See* Mediastinum and hila
HRCT patterns
  ground-glass opacities, 112–114
  peribronchovascular interstitial thickening, 117–118
  septal thickening, 115–116
  small nodular opacities, 119–122

small nodule distribution, 123–125
Hydronephrosis, 260, 268
Hyperalimentation, 224
Hyperinflation, compensatory, 48
Hyperlucent lung, 48–49
  unilateral, 49
Hyperparathyroidism, 265
Hyperplasia, 253
Hypersensitivity pneumonitis, 115
Hypertension, 179
Hypertrophy, kidney, 260
Hypervascular liver lesion, 219–220
  benign tumors, 219–220
  malignant tumors, 219
Hypervascular lymph nodes, 9
Hypervascular pancreatic mass, 249

# I

Iatrogenic pneumothorax, 128
Ileus, 290–291, 301
Infantile polycystic disease, 274
Infection
  gastrointestinal tract, 294–295
  ground-glass HRCT opacities, 113–114
  low-attenuation adenopathy, 7
  nodular interstitial disease, 92
  small nodular opacities, 119–120
  splenomegaly, 235
Infectious pericarditis, 176
Inflammatory polyp, 229
Injection granulomata, 331
Interstitial lung disease
  diffuse, 88–90
    with adenopathy, 96–97
    with pleural efusion, 95
  nodular, 91–94
Intraabdominal inflammation, 291
Intrahepatic biliary dilatation, 226–227
Intussusception, 302
Ischemia
  gastrointestinal tract, 296
  kidney, 258–259
Ischemic heart disease, 172
Islet cell tumor, 249

# K

Kidneys
  bilateral large kidneys, 262–264
    inflammation, 263–264
    masses, 264
  bilateral small kidneys, 259

Kidneys (*Continued*):
    failure of, 30, 131, 139
    hydronephrosis, 268
    perinephric lesion, 277
    renal calcifications, 265–267
        cortical nephrocalcinosis, 266
        medullary nephrocalcinosis, 265–266
    renal cysts, 274–276
    renal mass, 269–272
    renal mass with fat, 273
    unilateral large kidney, 260–261
    unilateral small kidney (atrophy or hypoplasia), 258

## L

Larynx, narrowed (true cords or subglottic), 22
Left to right shunt, 180
Leiomyoma, 299
Leiomyomata (fibroids), 319
Leukemia, 96
Lipoma, 148, 299
Liver
    cyst, 217–218
    fatty liver, 204
    hepatic calcifications, 206–207
    hepatomegaly, 198–201
    high density liver precontrast, 205
    lesions, 208–210. *See also* Tumors
        benign tumors, 209–210
        with central scar, 221
        hypervascular, 219–220
        low density postcontrast, 215–216
        low density precontrast, 212–214
        malignant tumors, 208–209
        multiple, 211
    low-density liver precontrast, 202–203
    portal venous gas, 222
Lobar consolidation, chronic, 104–106
    recurrent pneumonia, 105–106
Loculated effusion, 144, 146
Low-attenuation adenopathy, 7–8
Low-attenuation mediastinal mass, 168–170
    fat density, 168
    fluid density, 168–170
    gastrointestinal, 170
Lower lung disease, 45–47
Lower neck and trachea
    cystic neck mass, 15–16
    enlarged parotid gland, 20–21

**INDEX** 355

   narrowed larynx (true cords
      or subglottic), 22
   neck mass, 12–14
   thoracic inlet or superior
      mediastinal mass, 17
   thyroid lesion, 18–19
   tracheal enlargement, 26
   tracheal narrowing, 23–25
   tracheal or endobronchial
      mass, 27
Lucent lesions or cysts, 69–71
Lung. *See also* "Pulmonary"
      entries
   abscess, 60, 65
   airspace disease
      chronic lobar
         consolidation,
         104–106
      diffuse pulmonary
         consolidation,
         107–109
      focal or multifocal
         consolidation, 98–101
      nodular pattern, 102–103
      pulmonary hemorrhage,
         110–111
   global pulmonary patterns
      asymmetric lung size, 50
      atelectasis and
         pulmonary collapse,
         51
      bronchiectasis, 52–53
      diffuse lung disease,
         30–37
      diffuse lung disease with
         normal or increased
         lung volumes, 38
      hyperlucent lung,
         48–49
      lower lung disease,
         45–47
      perihilar lung disease,
         41–42
      peripheral lung disease,
         39–40
      upper lung disease,
         43–44
   HRCT patterns
      ground-glass opacities,
         112–114
      peribronchovascular
         interstitial thickening,
         117–118
      septal thickening,
         115–116
      small nodular opacities,
         119–122
      small nodule distribution
         on HRCT, 123–125
   interstitial lung disease
      diffuse interstitial disease
         with adenopathy,
         96–97
      diffuse interstitial disease
         with pleural effusion,
         95
      diffuse interstitial lung
         disease, 88–90
      nodular interstitial
         disease, 91–94

Lung (*Continued*):
  pulmonary cysts and nodules
    calcified pulmonary nodules, 86–87
    cavitary lung lesion, 65–68
    lucent lesions or cysts, 69–71
    multiple cavitary nodules, 79–81
    multiple ill-defined pulmonary nodules, 76–78
    multiple well-defined pulmonary nodules, 72–75
    peripheral pulmonary mass, 63–64
    pulmonary nodules with adenopathy, 85
    solitary pulmonary mass, 59–62
    solitary pulmonary nodule, 54–58
    tiny nodules, 82–84
  size, asymmetric, 50
Lymphadenopathy, 161–162, 191
Lymphangitic carcinomatosis, 88, 92, 115, 120, 123
Lymph nodes
  dimensions, 4
  enlarged. *See* Adenopathy
Lymphoma, 13, 17, 96, 144, 157, 161, 191, 194, 235, 237, 284, 286, 295, 299
Lytic bone lesion, 335–336

## M

Mediastinum and hila
  anterior mediastinal mass, 157–159
  cardiophrenic angle mass, 155–156
  hilar enlargement
    bilateral, 153–154
    unilateral, 151–152
  low attenuation mediastinal mass, 168–170
  middle mediastinal mass, 160–164
  pneumomediastinum, 150
  posterior mediastinal mass, 165–167
Medullary sponge kidney, 265
Mesenteric mass, 191–192
Micronodular disease. *See* Tiny nodules
Middle mediastinal mass, 160–164
  lymphadenopathy, 161–162
  primary tumors, 162–163
  vascular, 160–161
Miliary disease. *See* Tiny nodules
Mitral annulus, 177

Mucinous cystadenoma carcinoma, 323
Multifocal consolidation, 98–101
  infection, 98–99
Multiple cavitary nodules, 79–81
  inflammatory, 79
  tumor, 79–80
Multiple ill-defined pulmonary nodules, 76–78
  infection, 76
  tumor, 76
  vascular, 77
Multiple liver lesions, 211
Multiple myeloma, 148, 335
Multiple well-defined pulmonary nodules, 72–75
  granulomatous disease, 72
  tumors, 72–73
  vascular, 73–74
Mycobacterial infection, 119, 125
Mycoplasma, 32

# N

Narrowed cecum, 308–309
  infection, 308–309
  inflammation, 308
  tumors, 309
Narrowed esophagus, 282–283
  esophagitis, 282
  tumors, 282–283
Narrowed larynx (true cords or subglottic), 22
Narrowed stomach, 284–285
Neck. *See* Lower neck and trachea
Necrotic adenopathy, 15
Necrotizing pneumonia, 65
Nephrolithiasis, 265
Neuroblastoma, 252, 254
Neurogenic tumor, 165
Nodules, pulmonary. *See* Lung, pulmonary cysts and nodules
Noncardiogenic edema, 107–108
Nondistended bladder, 313

# O

Obesity, fatty liver and, 204
Obstruction
  kidney, 260
  ureter, 312
  uterus, 319
Opportunistic infections, 33–34
Organized pneumonia, 60, 63
Outlet (bladder) obstruction, 313

Ovaries
  calcified lesion, 326
  mass
    cystic, 324–325
    solid, 321–323
Ovulation, 318

## P

Pancreas
  calcification, 243–244
  cyst, 245
  fatty change, 242
  mass, 226, 246–248
    hypervascular, 249
Pancreatitis, 187, 284, 293
  chronic, 243
Parapelvic cysts, 274
Parapneumonic effusion, 132, 135–136
Parotid gland, enlarged, 20–21
Pelvic fluid (cul-de-sac), 318
Penetrating injury, 150
Peptic gastritis, 284
Perforated bowel, 184
Perforated stomach, 184
Peribronchovascular interstitial thickening, 117–118
Pericardial cyst, 155, 168
Pericardial effusion, 140–141, 176
Pericardial fat, 155

Perihilar lung disease, 41–42
Perinephric abscess, 277
Perinephric lesion, 277
Peripheral lung disease, 39–40, 144
Peripheral pulmonary mass, 63–64
Peritoneum
  abdominal abscess, 187–188
  ascites, 185–186
  peritoneal lesion, 189–190
  pneumoperitoneum, 184
Peritonitis, 290
Phrenic nerve paralysis, 50
PID, 324
Pleura
  calcifications, 143
  effusion. *See* Pleural effusion
  extrapleural lesion, 148
  fluid, types of, 131–134
    chylothorax, 133–134
    exudate, 132
    hemothorax, 133
    transudate, 131–132
  mass, 144–145
    multiple, 146–147
    neoplasm, 144–145
  plaques, 144, 146
  pneumothorax, 128–130
  thickening of, 142, 144
Pleural effusion
  bilateral, 138–139
    abdominal disease, 139

with cardiomegaly,
 140–141
 associated pericardial
  effusion, 140–141
 diffuse interstitial disease
  with, 95
 unilateral, 135–137
  cardiovascular, 135
  inflammatory, 135–136
  malignancy, 136
  traumatic, 137
Pneumatoceles, 48, 69
Pneumatosis intestinalis,
 288–289
Pneumobilia, 222, 231
Pneumomediastinum, 150
Pneumonia, 31–32, 39, 45,
 52, 54, 60, 88, 104
 *Pneumocystis carinii*
  pneumonia, 33, 113,
  129–130
Pneumoperitoneum, 184
Pneumothorax
 diffuse lung disease,
  129–130
 focal lung disease, 128–129
 pleural, 130
 trauma, 128
Polycystic disease, 274
Portal venous gas, 222
Posterior mediastinal mass,
 165–167
 gastrointestinal, 166
 paraspinal, 167
 spinal mass, 165–166

vascular, 167
Postobstructive atrophy,
 kidney, 258
Postobstructive infection,
 99
Postobstructive pneumonia,
 104
Postoperative abdominal
 abscess, 187
Prostate, enlarged, 305
Pseudocyst, 245, 248
Pseudomembranous colitis,
 303
Pulmonary artery
 hilar enlargement and,
  152–153
 hypertension of, 180
Pulmonary collapse, 50–51
Pulmonary consolidation,
 diffuse, 107–109
Pulmonary contusion, 110
Pulmonary cysts and nodules.
 *See* Lung, pulmonary
  cysts and nodules
Pulmonary edema, 30–31, 88,
 95, 107, 112, 115, 117
Pulmonary embolism, 135
Pulmonary fibrosis, 26, 39,
 45–46, 91, 115
Pulmonary hemorrhage, 108,
 110–111, 120
Pulmonary patterns, global.
 *See* Lung, global
  pulmonary patterns
Pulmonary resection, 50

Pulmonary venous hypertension, 180
Pyelonephritis, 260

## R

Radiation, 313
Recurrent pneumonia, 105–106
Reflux, 282
Renal calcifications, 265–267
Renal cell carcinoma, 269, 277
Renal cysts, 265, 269, 274–276
Renal failure, 30, 131, 139
Renal mass, 269–272
   with fat, 273
Renal osteodystrophy, 337
Renal tubular acidosis, 265
Retroperitoneum
   fibrosis, 193
   mass, 194–195
Right ventricular failure, 174
Rounded atelectasis, 57, 61, 63
Round pneumonia, 54, 60
Ruptured cystic airspace, 128

## S

Sarcoidosis, 83, 85, 96, 102, 117, 121, 123, 153
Scleroderma, 331
Sclerosing cholangitis, 226
Sclerotic bone lesion, 333–334
Sebaceous cyst, 329
Seminal vesicles and vas deferens, calcified, 317
Septal thickening, 115–116
Septic emboli, 77, 79
Serous cystadenoma carcinoma, 321
Sickle cell disease, 240, 337
Silicosis, 5, 83
Small bowel
   dilated, 290–292
   mass, 299–300
   thickened, 293–296
Small nodular opacities (HRCT), 119–122
Small nodule distribution (HRCT), 123–125
   centrilobular, 124–125
   perilymphatic, 123–124
   randomly distributed, 124
Soft tissue calcifications, 331–332
Solitary pulmonary mass, 59–62
   inflammatory, 60–61
   tumor, 59
Solitary pulmonary nodule, 54–58
   inflammatory, 54–55
   neoplasm, 55–56
   vascular, 56–57

Sphincterotomy, 231
Spinal mass, 165–166
Spleen
  calcifications, 240
  cyst, 239
  lesion, 237–238
  small, 234
  splenomegaly, 235–236
  splenule, 234
Steroids, fatty liver and, 204
Stomach, 156, 166, 170
  gastric mass, 286–287
  perforated, 184
  thickened or narrowed, 284–285
Stromal tumors (ovaries), 322
Superior mediastinal mass, 17
Surgery, prior, 138, 150, 184, 225, 290

# T

Thickened colon, 303–305
  inflammation, 303–304
  tumors, 304
Thickened or narrowed stomach, 284–285
  inflammation, 284–285
  tumors, 284
Thickened small bowel, 293–296
  edema, 293
  infection/enteritis, 294–295
  inflammation, 293–294
  tumors, 295
Thickened terminal ileum, 297–298
  infection, 297
  inflammation, 297
  tumors, 298
Thoracic duct, traumatic injury to, 133
Thoracic inlet mass, 17
Thymic mass, 157
Thyroid lesion, 18–19
Thyroid mass, 17, 157
Tiny nodules, 82–84
  inflammatory, 82
  malignancy, 83
Trachea. *See* Lower neck and trachea
Tracheomalacia, 26
Traction bronchiectasis, 52
Transitional cell carcinoma, 269
Transudate, 131–132
Trauma
  chest and abdominal wall, 133, 331
  genitourinary tract, 316
  liver cyst, 217
  lung, 110
  mediastinum, 150
  pneumothorax and, 128
  tracheal narrowing, 23
  unilateral pleural effusion, 137
Tuboovarian abscess, 324

Tumors. *See also* names of
specific tumors (e.g.,
Adenocarcinoma;
Hamartoma; etc.)
adrenal glands, 252–254
body wall, 329
bone, 335
cardiac, 175
colon, 304
esophagus, 282–283
kidney, 260, 269–271
larynx, 22
liver, 198–199, 206–213, 215, 219–220
lung, 34, 119–122
mediastinum and hila, 162–163
neck, 13
ovaries, 321–323
pancreas, 243, 245–247
small bowel, 295, 299–300
spleen, 237
stomach, 284, 286
terminal ileum, 298

## U

Ulcerative colitis, 303
Unilateral large kidney, 260–261
Unilateral small kidney (atrophy or hypoplasia), 258
UPJ obstruction, 268
Upper lung disease, 43–44
Ureteral dilatation, 312
Ureteral obstruction, 268
Uterus, enlarged, 319–320

## V

Vascular calcifications, 243
Vascular diagnoses. *See* Cardiac and vascular diagnoses
Vas deferens and seminal vesicles, calcified, 317
Vesicoureteral reflux, 312
Viral infection, 113
Vocal cord paralysis, 22
Volotrauma, 128, 150

## W

Wegener granulomatosis, 73, 77
Wilms tumor, 269

## X

Xanthogranulomatous pyelonephritis, 273

ISBN 0-07-134435-7